ISBN: 9781080988853

WEIGHT LOSS
For Men
Metric Edition

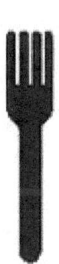

My Calendar

S	M	T	W	Th	F	S
				1	2	3
4	5	6	7	8	9	10
11	12	13	14	15	16	17
18	19	20	21	22	23	24
25	26	27	28	29	30	

Vincent Antonetti, Ph.D.

NoPaperPress.com™

TABLE OF CONTENTS

Disclaimer

LIST OF TABLES

1. BEFORE YOU BEGIN

Most people in industrialized countries are far less physically active than their counterparts of a few generations ago. But their caloric intake has not decreased proportionately. In fact, enough food is produced in the United States to supply 3,800 Calories per day to every man, woman and child – far more than anyone needs. As a result more people than ever suffer from excess weight, and the problems and health risks that accompany being overweight or obese. In the United States, recent estimates indicate more than 40 million people are obese!

Being overweight or obese matters. Excess weight puts undo strain on your body. Studies have shown that overweight people have a greater risk of serious illness than those who are slimmer – and the greater the degree of overweight the greater the risk. People who are overweight are more susceptible to certain illnesses, especially heart and circulatory diseases, type-2 diabetes, as well as gallbladder and liver disorders. Being overweight also has a negative impact on self esteem and appearance

To millions of people losing weight has become not only a goal but almost a way of life. The fact that so many have found it difficult to realize their aspiration has fostered a flood of fad diet books. Some of the diets insist that it's not how much you eat but the combination of foods, or the type of food you eat that's important. Most exclude forbidden (but often nutritious and reasonably low calorie) foods. Others are big on motivation and offer hand-holding emotional support but little else. In fact, almost every diet book on the market is devoid of hard facts, real data, analysis and insight.

The truth is that weight control, although a relatively complex issue, is governed by a set of logical, scientific principles, and the acceptance and understanding of these principles – augmented of course by desire and self-discipline – can lead you to sure and lasting weight management. Concerning weight control, Lori Love, M.D., Ph.D., formerly of the United States Food and Drug Administration's Center for Food Safety and Applied Nutrition, states, "There are no shortcuts – no magic pills."

Most health professional agree that losing weight sensibly and safely requires a multifaceted approach that includes setting reasonable weight-loss goals, changing eating habits, and getting adequate exercise.

Long-term success is not about finding the "right" diet. It's about developing both an understanding and a plan that will result in healthier eating and physical activity habits. Without a doubt identifying the behaviors that have contributed to your eating more calories than your body needs is important, very important. But assuming you are successful in determining why you overeat, what do you do next? The desire to lose weight and the discipline to start and stay on a weight-control program are crucial. But along with desire and discipline, it is our belief that **only an in-depth understanding of weight control, nutrition and exercise will lead to long-term success**. As is true with many important and complex subjects, to achieve you need more than rules – you need information and a solid understanding. We leave behavioral analysis and motivation to others. Our mission is to impart facts, data, knowledge and the systematic approach needed for enduring weight management. So take the time to read what follows. The reward will last you a lifetime.

Start with a Medical Exam: Everyone should have a medical assessment, or exam, before starting a weight control and/or physical fitness program. You need to make sure your health will allow you to lower your caloric intake and increase your physical activity. The medical checkup may be as simple as a visit to a physician who is familiar with your medical history, or it may be a thorough physical exam. Note, in all cases the physician conducting the medical exam should be made aware of and should approve the specific weight management and/or physical fitness program you are planning.

What Should You Weigh?

Recently, many health-care practitioners rely on Body Mass Index, or BMI, to determine if a person is overweight. The BMI takes into account both a person's weight and height and is calculated by dividing a person's weight in kilograms by the square of their height (in meters). For readers living in the United States, Table 1 provides a convenient determination of BMI, using body weight in pounds and height in feet and inches. This table is not applicable to competitive athletes, body builders and the chronically ill.

The rationale behind the BMI is based on epidemiological data that show an increase in mortality when the BMI is above 25, although the increase in mortality tends to be moderate until a BMI of 30 is reached. Table 2 (on the next page) shows how scientists categorize a person's body-weight as a function of their BMI.

Weight (kg.)	- Height (cm.) -									
	155	160	165	170	175	180	185	190	195	200
45	18.7	17.6								
50	20.8	19.5	18.4							
55	22.9	21.5	20.2	19.0	18.0					
60	25.0	23.4	22.0	20.8	19.6	18.5	17.5			
65	27.1	25.4	23.9	22.5	21.2	20.2	19.0	18.0		
70	29.1	27.3	25.7	24.2	22.9	21.6	20.5	19.4	18.4	17.5
75	31.2	29.3	27.5	26.0	24.5	23.1	21.9	20.8	19.7	18.8
80	33.3	31.2	29.4	27.7	26.1	24.7	23.4	22.2	21.0	20.0
90	37.5	35.2	33.1	31.1	29.4	27.8	26.3	24.9	23.7	22.5
100	41.6	39.1	36.7	34.6	32.7	30.9	29.2	27.7	26.3	25.0
120	49.9	46.9	44.1	41.5	39.2	37.0	35.1	33.2	31.6	30.0
140			51.4	48.4	45.7	43.2	40.9	38.8	36.8	35.0
160				55.4	52.2	49.4	46.7	44.3	42.1	40.0
180						55.6	52.6	49.9	47.3	45.0

Table 1 Body Mass Index (BMI)

BMI	Weight Profile
18.5 or less	Underweight
18.6 to 24.9	Normal
25.0 to 29.9	Overweight
30.0 to 39.9	Obese
40 or more	Extremely Obese

Table 2 Weight Profile vs. BMI

BMI-Based Weight vs. Height

Another more convenient way to use BMI is the New BMI-Based Weight vs. Height Chart shown in Table 3, where normal weight is for BMI = 18.6 to 24.9, overweight is for BMI = 25.0 to 29.9,and obese is for BMI = 30.0 to 39.9.

Table 3 BMI-Based Weight vs. Height

Height (cm)	Normal Range	Overweight Range	Obese Range
150	41.9 – 56.0	56.1 – 67.3	67.4 – 89.8
152	43.0 – 57.5	57.6 – 69.1	69.2 – 92.2
154	44.1 – 59.1	59.2 – 70.9	71.0 – 94.6
156	45.3 – 60.6	60.7 – 72.8	72.9 – 97.1
158	46.4 – 62.2	62.3 – 74.6	74.7 – 99.6
160	47.6 – 63.7	63.8 – 76.5	76.6 – 102.1
162	48.8 – 65.3	65.4 – 78.5	78.6 – 104.7
164	50.0 – 67.0	67.1 – 80.4	80.5 – 107.3
166	51.3 – 68.6	68.7 – 82.4	82.5 – 109.9
168	52.5 – 70.3	70.4 – 84.4	84.5 – 112.6
170	53.8 – 72.0	72.1 – 86.4	86.5 – 115.3
172	55.0 – 73.7	73.8 – 88.5	88.6 – 118.0
174	56.3 – 75.4	75.5 – 90.5	90.6 – 120.8
176	57.6 – 77.1	77.2 – 92.6	92.7 – 123.6
178	58.9 – 78.9	79.0 – 94.7	94.8 – 126.4
180	60.3 – 80.7	80.8 – 96.9	97.0 – 129.3
182	61.6 – 82.5	82.6 – 99.0	99.1 – 132.2
184	63.0 – 84.3	84.4 – 101.2	101.3 – 135.1
186	64.3 – 86.1	86.2 – 103.4	103.5 – 138.0
188	65.7 – 88.0	88.1 – 105.7	105.8 – 141.0
190	67.1 – 89.9	90.0 – 107.9	108.0 – 144.0
192	68.6 – 91.8	91.9 – 110.2	110.3 – 147.1
194	70.0 – 93.7	93.8 – 112.5	112.6 – 150.2
196	71.5 – 95.7	95.8 – 114.9	115.0 – 153.3
198	72.9 – 97.6	97.7 – 117.2	117.3 – 156.4
200	74.4 – 99.6	99.7 – 119.6	119.7 – 159.6

Example: Determine BMI of a man who is 190 cm tall and weighs 80 kg. First use Table 1. Scan the far left of the table and locate his weight of 80 kg. From this number run your finger horizontally (to the right) until it intersects the vertical column headed by his 190 cm height. The number at the intersection is his BMI = 22.2. According to Table 2 his weight is in the normal range.

Example: Determine the normal weight range for a man who is 190 cm tall. From Table 3, find that at 190 cm he must weigh between 67.1 and 89.9 kg for his weight to be in the "normal" range, that is for his BMI to be between 18.6 and 24.9. (I think you will agree that the information provided by Table 3 is more useful than that provided by Table 1.)

Body Fat Storage

Many health care professionals contend that overweight or obesity does not depend on body weight but on the amount of body fat compared to total body weight. Body fat exists in two storage sites. The first storage depot, consists of the intestines, muscles, and the lipid-rich tissues throughout the central nervous system. This is referred to as Essential Fat and is required, or essential is necessary to maintain health. In females, essential fat also includes sex-specific or sex-characteristic fat. The average man requires approximately 3% essential fat, and the average woman about 10%. The higher percentage of essential fat in females includes about 7% of sex-specific fat, believed to be important for child-bearing and other hormone-related functions.

The other major fat type is called storage fat and consists of fat that accumulates in adipose tissue. The main function of adipose tissue is to store energy in the form of fat which can be used to meet the energy needs of the body. Adipose tissue also cushions and insulates the body and serves as an important endocrine organ by producing needed hormones. The formation of adipose tissue appears to be controlled by an adipose gene. Adipose tissue is found in specific locations, which are referred to as "adipose depots," located beneath the skin (subcutaneous fat), around internal organs (visceral fat), in bone marrow (yellow bone marrow) and in breast tissue. Female sex hormones cause fat to be stored in the buttocks, thighs, and hips in women; whereas, men are more likely to have fat stored in the belly.

Percent Body Fat

Lean body weight consists of all the non-fat tissue such as muscle, bone, organs and connective tissue. The remainder is the fat component and is most often expressed as a percentage of total body weight, represented as "body fat percentage." Exercise physiologists consider the quantity of body fat compared to total body weight a critical measure of fitness and much more important than a person's actual weight. An age-adjusted weight profile for men versus body fat percentage is shown in Table 4 on the following page.

Age	Underweight	Healthy	Overweight	Obese
21 - 40	8 % or less	8 - 19 %	19 - 25 %	Over 25%
41 - 60	11% or less	11 - 22 %	22 - 27 %	Over 27%
61 - 80	13% or less	13 - 25 %	25 - 30 %	Over 30%

Table 4 Age-Adjusted Body Fat Percentage
Source: Gallagher et al., Am J Clin Nut 2000; 72:694-701

Measuring Percent Body Fat

There are several methods for assessing body composition and fat percentage. The most common are underwater weighing, DEXA, bioelectrical impedance, skin-fold measurements and body-girth measurements.

Body-Girth Measurements: Lately, obesity researchers have shown that body girth measurements at three or four locations (along with a correlating equation) can be used to estimate percent body fat with a reasonable degree of accuracy. For men body fat percentage is dependent on waist and neck circumferences as well as height. This body-fat percentage assessment technique is simple, fast, inexpensive (requires no special tools) and can be performed in an office. As with the skin-fold technique, there are two ways to use this method. The first is to use the sum of the measurements and the second is to use the measurements in conjunction with the correlation developed by the U.S. Naval Health Research Center* to predict fat percentage. The Body-Girth method is what we at NoPaperPress prefer and advocate because we believe it to be reasonably accurate and the most practical.

* Source: Hodgdon, J.A. and Beckett, M.B. (1984b). Prediction of percent body fat for U.S. Navy women from body circumferences and height. Report No. 84-11, Naval Health Research Center, San Diego, CA

Percent Body Fat Table

For this book, the U.S. Navy body-girth correlation equation was used to develop Table 5 (on page 15), a body fat percentage table for men. The value of putting the data in tabular form is that it allows a user to understand how changes in MP (male parameter) affect body fat percentage.

Example: Determine the percent body fat of a 47 year-old man, 170 cm tall, whose body girth was measured as follows:

Waist circumference = 86 cm

Hip circumference = 92 cm

Neck circumference = 40 cm

First, calculate the Male Parameter (MP) which is equal to the man's waist circumference minus his neck circumference, or MP = 86 – 40 = 46

Now enter the left column of Table 5 with MP = 46. From this number run your finger horizontally (to the right) until it intersects the vertical column headed by his 180 cm height. The number at the intersection is his Body Fat Percentage = 15.3 %.

According to Table 4, a healthy body fat percentage range for men ages 41 to 60 is 11 to 22 %. Thus at 15.3 % this 47 year-old man's body fat percentage is in the healthy range.

Waist to Hip Ratio

The waist-to-hip ratio is often viewed as an indicator of health and the risk of developing serious health conditions. It is also used as a measurement of obesity, which in turn is a possible indicator of other more serious health conditions.

Measurement: The waist is measured at the smallest circumference of your natural waist, usually just above the belly button. If the waist is convex rather than concave, such as is the case in obesity, the waist should be measured at a horizontal level one-inch above the navel. Hip circumference is measured at the widest part of the buttocks or hip.

Health risks for heart attack and stroke increase considerably for men with a ratio above 1.0 and for women with a ratio above 0.8. A ratio of .90 or less in men correlates strongly with general health and fertility. Men with a ratio around 0.9 are generally healthier and more fertile with less prostate and testicular cancer.

Example: Calculate the waist-to-hip ratio for the man in the previous example. Recall his measurements were as follows: Waist circumference = 86 cm, Hip circumference = 92 cm. Hence his Waist-to-Hip Ratio = 86 / 92 = 0.93, which is good.

Table 5 Approx Percent Body Fat

MP	HEIGHT (cm)									
	155	160	165	170	175	180	185	190	195	200
36	10.7	9.8	8.8							
38	12.8	11.8	10.9	10.0	9.1					
40	14.7	13.7	12.8	11.9	11.0	10.1	9.3			
42	16.5	15.5	14.6	13.7	12.8	12.0	11.1	10.3	9.5	
44	18.2	17.3	16.3	15.4	14.5	13.7	12.9	12.0	11.3	10.5
46	19.9	18.9	18.0	17.1	16.2	15.3	14.5	13.7	12.9	12.1
48	21.5	20.5	19.6	18.7	17.8	16.9	16.1	15.3	14.5	13.7
50	23.0	22.0	21.1	20.2	19.3	18.5	17.6	16.8	16.0	15.3
52	24.5	23.5	22.6	21.7	20.8	19.9	19.1	18.3	17.5	16.7
54	25.9	24.9	24.0	23.1	22.2	21.3	20.5	19.7	18.9	18.1
56	27.2	26.3	25.3	24.4	23.6	22.7	21.9	21.1	20.3	19.5
58	28.6	27.6	26.7	25.7	24.9	24.0	23.2	22.4	21.6	20.8
60	29.8	28.9	27.9	27.0	26.1	25.3	24.4	23.6	22.8	22.1
62	31.0	30.1	29.1	28.2	27.4	26.5	25.7	24.9	24.1	23.3
64	32.2	31.3	30.3	29.4	28.5	27.7	26.9	26.0	25.3	24.5
66	33.4	32.4	31.5	30.6	29.7	28.8	28.0	27.2	26.4	25.6
68	34.5	33.5	32.6	31.7	30.8	29.9	29.1	28.3	27.5	26.7
70	35.6	34.6	33.7	32.8	31.9	31.0	30.2	29.4	28.6	27.8
72	36.6	35.7	34.7	33.8	32.9	32.1	31.3	30.4	29.6	28.9
74		36.7	35.8	34.8	34.0	33.1	32.3	31.5	30.7	29.9
76			36.8	35.8	35.0	34.1	33.3	32.5	31.7	30.9
78				36.8	35.9	35.1	34.2	33.4	32.6	31.9
80					36.9	36.0	35.2	34.4	33.6	32.8
82						36.9	36.1	35.3	34.5	33.7
84							37.0	36.2	35.4	34.6

FP = Waist Circumference – Neck Circumference (cm)

Maximum Waist Size

The waist size beyond which a man has increased health risk is referred to as his maximum waist size.   To determine maximum waist size, a maximum waist-to-hip ratio of 1.0 was inserted into the U.S. Navy body-girth correlation equation and a maximum age adjusted body fat percentage was used from Table 4 on page 13. (For example, for men 20 to 40 years old a body fat percentage of 19% was used.) From this a maximum waist size was determined as a function of neck size and height. The resulting equation is presented in tabular form in Tables 6 to 8 on pages 17 to 19.

Example: Determine the maximum waist size for the 29 year-old man whose is 180 cm tall and has a 40-cm neck circumference.
Enter the left column of Table 6 with a height of 180 cm. From this number run your finger horizontally (to the right) until it intersects the vertical column headed by his 40-cm neck size. The number at the intersection is his Maximum Waist Size which is 90.7 cm.

Table 6 Max Waist - Ages 20 to 40

Height (cm)	NECK SIZE (cm)									
	37	38	39	40	41	42	43	44	45	46
156	82.1	83.1	84.1	85.1	86.1	87.1	88.1	89.1	90.1	91.1
158	82.6	83.6	84.6	85.6	86.6	87.6	88.6	89.6	90.6	91.6
160	83.1	84.1	85.1	86.1	87.1	88.1	89.1	90.1	91.1	92.1
162	83.5	84.5	85.5	86.5	87.5	88.5	89.5	90.5	91.5	92.5
164	84.0	85.0	86.0	87.0	88.0	89.0	90.0	91.0	92.0	93.0
166	84.5	85.5	86.5	87.5	88.5	89.5	90.5	91.5	92.5	93.5
168	84.9	85.9	86.9	87.9	88.9	89.9	90.9	91.9	92.9	93.9
170	85.4	86.4	87.4	88.4	89.4	90.4	91.4	92.4	93.4	94.4
172	85.8	86.8	87.8	88.8	89.8	90.8	91.8	92.8	93.8	94.8
174	86.3	87.3	88.3	89.3	90.3	91.3	92.3	93.3	94.3	95.3
176	86.8	87.8	88.8	89.8	90.8	91.8	92.8	93.8	94.8	95.8
178	87.2	88.2	89.2	90.2	91.2	92.2	93.2	94.2	95.2	96.2
180	87.7	88.7	89.7	**90.7**	91.7	92.7	93.7	94.7	95.7	96.7
182	88.1	89.1	90.1	91.1	92.1	93.1	94.1	95.1	96.1	97.1
184	88.6	89.6	90.6	91.6	92.6	93.6	94.6	95.6	96.6	97.6
186	89.1	90.1	91.1	92.1	93.1	94.1	95.1	96.1	97.1	98.1
188	89.5	90.5	91.5	92.5	93.5	94.5	95.5	96.5	97.5	98.5
190	90.0	91.0	92.0	93.0	94.0	95.0	96.0	97.0	98.0	99.0
192	90.4	91.4	92.4	93.4	94.4	95.4	96.4	97.4	98.4	99.4
194	90.9	91.9	92.9	93.9	94.9	95.9	96.9	97.9	98.9	99.9
196	91.3	92.3	93.3	94.3	95.3	96.3	97.3	98.3	99.3	100.3
198	91.8	92.8	93.8	94.8	95.8	96.8	97.8	98.8	99.8	100.8
200	92.2	93.2	94.2	95.2	96.2	97.2	98.2	99.2	100.2	101.2

Values in table are waist size (cm)

Table 7 Max Waist - Ages 41 to 60

Height (cm)	NECK SIZE (cm)									
	37	38	39	40	41	42	43	44	45	46
156	85.9	86.9	87.9	88.9	89.9	90.9	91.9	92.9	93.9	94.9
158	86.4	87.4	88.4	89.4	90.4	91.4	92.4	93.4	94.4	95.4
160	86.9	87.9	88.9	89.9	90.9	91.9	92.9	93.9	94.9	95.9
162	87.4	88.4	89.4	90.4	91.4	92.4	93.4	94.4	95.4	96.4
164	87.9	88.9	89.9	90.9	91.9	92.9	93.9	94.9	95.9	96.9
166	88.4	89.4	90.4	91.4	92.4	93.4	94.4	95.4	96.4	97.4
168	88.9	89.9	90.9	91.9	92.9	93.9	94.9	95.9	96.9	97.9
170	89.4	90.4	91.4	92.4	93.4	94.4	95.4	96.4	97.4	98.4
172	89.9	90.9	91.9	92.9	93.9	94.9	95.9	96.9	97.9	98.9
174	90.4	91.4	92.4	93.4	94.4	95.4	96.4	97.4	98.4	99.4
176	90.9	91.9	92.9	93.9	94.9	95.9	96.9	97.9	98.9	99.9
178	91.4	92.4	93.4	94.4	95.4	96.4	97.4	98.4	99.4	100.4
180	91.9	92.9	93.9	94.9	95.9	96.9	97.9	98.9	99.9	100.9
182	92.4	93.4	94.4	95.4	96.4	97.4	98.4	99.4	100.4	101.4
184	92.9	93.9	94.9	95.9	96.9	97.9	98.9	99.9	100.9	101.9
186	93.4	94.4	95.4	96.4	97.4	98.4	99.4	100.4	101.4	102.4
188	93.9	94.9	95.9	96.9	97.9	98.9	99.9	100.9	101.9	102.9
190	94.4	95.4	96.4	97.4	98.4	99.4	100.4	101.4	102.4	103.4
192	94.9	95.9	96.9	97.9	98.9	99.9	100.9	101.9	102.9	103.9
194	95.4	96.4	97.4	98.4	99.4	100.4	101.4	102.4	103.4	104.4
196	95.9	96.9	97.9	98.9	99.9	100.9	101.9	102.9	103.9	104.9
198	96.4	97.4	98.4	99.4	100.4	101.4	102.4	103.4	104.4	105.4
200	96.8	97.8	98.8	99.8	100.8	101.8	102.8	103.8	104.8	104.8

Values in table are waist size (cm)

Table 8 Max Waist - Ages 61 to 80

Height (cm)	NECK SIZE (cm)									
	37	38	39	40	41	42	43	44	45	46
156	90.0	91.0	92.0	93.0	94.0	95.0	96.0	97.0	98.0	99.0
158	90.5	91.5	92.5	93.5	94.5	95.5	96.5	97.5	98.5	99.5
160	91.1	92.1	93.1	94.1	95.1	96.1	97.1	98.1	99.1	100.1
162	91.6	92.6	93.6	94.6	95.6	96.6	97.6	98.6	99.6	100.6
164	92.2	93.2	94.2	95.2	96.2	97.2	98.2	99.2	100.2	101.2
166	92.7	93.7	94.7	95.7	96.7	97.7	98.7	99.7	100.7	101.7
168	93.3	94.3	95.3	96.3	97.3	98.3	99.3	100.3	101.3	102.3
170	93.8	94.8	95.8	96.8	97.8	98.8	99.8	100.8	101.8	102.8
172	94.4	95.4	96.4	97.4	98.4	99.4	100.4	101.4	102.4	103.4
174	94.9	95.9	96.9	97.9	98.9	99.9	100.9	101.9	102.9	103.9
176	95.4	96.4	97.4	98.4	99.4	100.4	101.4	102.4	103.4	104.4
178	96.0	97.0	98.0	99.0	100.0	101.0	102.0	103.0	104.0	105.0
180	96.5	97.5	98.5	99.5	100.5	101.5	102.5	103.5	104.5	105.5
182	97.1	98.1	99.1	100.1	101.1	102.1	103.1	104.1	105.1	106.1
184	97.6	98.6	99.6	100.6	101.6	102.6	103.6	104.6	105.6	106.6
186	98.1	99.1	100.1	101.1	102.1	103.1	104.1	105.1	106.1	107.1
188	98.7	99.7	100.7	101.7	102.7	103.7	104.7	105.7	106.7	107.7
190	99.2	100.2	101.2	102.2	103.2	104.2	105.2	106.2	107.2	108.2
192	99.7	100.7	101.7	102.7	103.7	104.7	105.7	106.7	107.7	108.7
194	100.3	101.3	102.3	103.3	104.3	105.3	106.3	107.3	108.3	109.3
196	100.8	101.8	102.8	103.8	104.8	105.8	106.8	107.8	108.8	109.8
198	101.3	102.3	103.3	104.3	105.3	106.3	107.3	108.3	109.3	110.3
200	101.9	102.9	103.9	104.9	105.9	106.9	107.9	108.9	109.9	110.9

Values in table are waist size (cm)

Optimum Waist Size

An optimum waist size is one that is strongly associated with general health. To determine optimum waist size, a healthier waist-to-hip ratio of 0.9 and a healthier age-adjusted body fat percentage from Table 4. (For example, for women 20 to 40 years old the average of 8 to 19 %, or 13.5 %

18

was used.) Then an optimum waist size as a function of neck size and height was determined. Again the unique resulting equation is arranged in tabular form in tables 9 to 11.

Example: Determine the optimum waist size for the 48 year-old man whose is 180 cm tall and has a 40 cm neck circumference.
Enter the left column of Table 10 with a height of 180 cm. From this number run your finger horizontally (to the right) until it intersects the vertical column headed by his 40 cm neck size. The number at the intersection is his Optimum Waist Size, which is 87.4 cm.

Table 9 Optimum Waist - Ages 20 to 40

Height (cm)	NECK SIZE (cm)									
	37	38	39	40	41	42	43	44	45	46
156	75.9	76.9	77.9	78.9	79.9	80.9	81.9	82.9	83.9	84.9
158	76.3	77.3	78.3	79.3	80.3	81.3	82.3	83.3	84.3	85.3
160	76.7	77.7	78.7	79.7	80.7	81.7	82.7	83.7	84.7	85.7
162	77.1	78.1	79.1	80.1	81.1	82.1	83.1	84.1	85.1	86.1
164	77.5	78.5	79.5	80.5	81.5	82.5	83.5	84.5	85.5	86.5
166	77.9	78.9	79.9	80.9	81.9	82.9	83.9	84.9	85.9	86.9
168	78.4	79.4	80.4	81.4	82.4	83.4	84.4	85.4	86.4	87.4
170	78.8	79.8	80.8	81.8	82.8	83.8	84.8	85.8	86.8	87.8
172	79.2	80.2	81.2	82.2	83.2	84.2	85.2	86.2	87.2	88.2
174	79.5	80.5	81.5	82.5	83.5	84.5	85.5	86.5	87.5	88.5
176	79.9	80.9	81.9	82.9	83.9	84.9	85.9	86.9	87.9	88.9
178	80.3	81.3	82.3	83.3	84.3	85.3	86.3	87.3	88.3	89.3
180	80.7	81.7	82.7	83.7	84.7	85.7	86.7	87.7	88.7	78.7
182	81.1	82.1	83.1	84.1	85.1	86.1	87.1	88.1	89.1	90.1
184	81.5	82.5	83.5	84.5	85.5	86.5	87.5	88.5	89.5	90.5
186	81.9	82.9	83.9	84.9	85.9	86.9	87.9	88.9	89.9	90.9
188	82.3	83.3	84.3	85.3	86.3	87.3	88.3	89.3	90.3	91.3
190	82.7	83.7	84.7	85.7	86.7	87.7	88.7	89.7	90.7	91.7
192	83.1	84.1	85.1	86.1	87.1	88.1	89.1	90.1	91.1	92.1
194	83.5	84.5	85.5	86.5	87.5	88.5	89.5	90.5	91.5	92.5
196	83.9	84.9	85.9	86.9	87.9	88.9	89.5	90.9	91.9	92.9
198	84.3	85.3	86.3	87.3	88.3	89.3	90.3	91.3	92.3	93.3
200	84.7	85.7	86.7	87.7	88.7	89.7	90.7	91.7	92.7	93.7

Values in table are waist size (cm)

Table 10 Optimum Waist - Ages 41 to 60

Height (cm)	NECK SIZE (cm)									
	37	38	39	40	41	42	43	44	45	46
156	79.2	80.2	81.2	82.2	83.2	84.2	85.2	86.2	87.2	88.2
158	79.6	80.6	81.6	82.6	83.6	84.6	85.6	86.6	87.6	88.6
160	80.1	81.1	82.1	83.1	84.1	85.1	86.1	87.1	88.1	89.1
162	80.5	81.5	82.5	83.5	84.5	85.5	86.5	87.5	88.5	89.5
164	80.9	81.9	82.9	83.9	84.9	85.9	86.9	87.9	88.9	89.9
166	81.4	82.4	83.4	84.4	85.4	86.4	87.4	88.4	89.4	90.4
168	81.8	82.8	83.8	84.8	85.8	86.8	87.8	88.8	89.8	90.8
170	82.2	83.2	84.2	85.2	86.2	87.2	88.2	89.2	90.2	91.2
172	82.7	83.7	84.7	85.7	86.7	87.7	88.7	89.7	90.7	91.7
174	83.1	84.1	85.1	86.1	87.1	88.1	89.1	90.1	91.1	92.1
176	83.5	84.5	85.5	86.5	87.5	88.5	89.5	90.5	91.5	92.5
178	84.0	85.0	86.0	87.0	88.0	89.0	90.0	91.0	92.0	93.0
180	84.4	85.4	86.4	**87.4**	88.4	89.4	90.4	91.4	92.4	93.4
182	84.8	85.8	86.8	87.8	88.8	89.8	90.8	91.8	92.8	93.8
184	85.3	86.3	87.3	88.3	89.3	90.3	91.3	92.3	94.3	95.3
186	85.7	86.7	87.7	88.7	89.7	90.7	91.7	92.7	93.7	94.7
188	86.1	87.1	88.1	89.1	90.1	91.1	92.1	93.1	94.1	95.1
190	86.5	87.5	88.5	89.5	90.5	91.5	92.5	93.5	94.5	95.5
192	87.0	88.0	89.0	90.0	91.0	92.0	93.0	94.0	95.0	96.0
194	87.4	88.4	89.4	90.4	91.4	92.4	93.4	94.4	95.4	96.4
196	87.8	88.8	89.8	90.8	91.8	92.8	93.8	94.8	95.8	96.8
198	88.2	89.2	90.2	91.2	92.2	93.2	94.2	95.2	96.2	97.2
200	88.6	89.6	90.6	91.6	92.6	93.6	94.6	95.6	96.6	97.6

Values in table are waist size (cm)

Table 11 Optimum Waist - Ages 61 to 80

Height (cm)	NECK SIZE (cm)									
	37	38	39	40	41	42	43	44	45	46
156	82.1	83.1	84.1	85.1	86.1	87.1	88.1	89.1	90.1	91.1
158	82.6	83.6	84.6	85.6	86.6	87.6	88.6	89.6	90.6	91.6
160	83.1	84.1	85.1	86.1	87.1	88.1	89.1	90.1	91.1	92.1
162	83.5	84.5	85.5	86.5	87.5	88.5	89.5	90.5	91.5	92.5
164	84.0	85.0	86.0	87.0	88.0	89.0	90.0	91.0	92.0	93.0
166	84.5	85.5	86.5	87.5	88.5	89.5	90.5	91.5	92.5	93.5
168	84.9	85.9	86.9	87.9	88.9	89.9	90.9	91.9	92.9	93.9
170	85.4	86.4	87.4	88.4	89.4	90.4	91.4	92.4	93.4	94.4
172	85.8	86.8	87.8	88.8	89.8	90.8	91.8	92.8	93.8	94.8
174	86.3	87.3	88.3	89.3	90.3	91.3	92.3	93.3	94.3	95.3
176	86.8	87.8	88.8	89.8	90.8	91.8	92.8	93.8	94.8	95.8
178	87.2	88.2	89.2	90.2	91.2	92.2	93.2	94.2	95.2	96.2
180	87.7	88.7	89.7	90.7	91.7	92.7	93.7	94.7	95.7	96.7
182	88.1	89.1	90.1	91.1	92.1	93.1	94.1	95.1	96.1	97.1
184	88.6	89.6	90.6	91.6	92.6	93.6	94.6	95.6	96.6	97.6
186	89.1	90.1	91.1	92.1	93.1	94.1	95.1	96.1	97.1	98.1
188	89.5	90.5	91.5	92.5	93.5	94.5	95.5	96.5	97.5	98.5
190	90.0	91.0	92.0	93.0	94.0	95.0	96.0	97.0	98.0	99.0
192	90.4	91.4	92.4	93.4	94.4	95.4	96.4	97.4	98.4	99.4
194	90.9	91.9	92.9	93.9	94.9	95.9	96.9	97.9	98.9	99.9
196	91.3	92.3	93.3	94.3	95.3	96.3	97.3	98.3	99.3	100.3
198	91.8	92.8	93.8	94.8	95.8	96.8	97.8	98.8	99.8	100.8
200	92.2	93.2	94.2	95.2	96.2	97.2	98.2	99.2	100.2	101.2

Values in table are waist size (cm)

2. WEIGHT LOSS

All human life depends on the energy that comes from the sun. Plants convert solar energy into chemical energy by photosynthesis. The chemical energy is then used by plants to make carbohydrates, proteins and fats. We need energy to operate our body, but we cannot use solar energy directly. Instead we get the energy we need from the chemical energy contained in plants or other animals. When we eat food containing carbohydrates, proteins and fats, they are oxidized producing energy, carbon dioxide, water – and heat. This chapter contains a brief discussion of energy, as it generally pertains to our bodies, and how energy relates to weight control.

Conservation of Energy

One of the greatest scientific achievements of the nineteenth century was the recognition and statement of the principle of conservation of energy by Julius Robert Von Mayer, in a classic paper written in 1842.. The principle is based on observation of physical phenomenon and states that energy may be converted or transferred but cannot be created or destroyed. Then in 1847, Von Helmholtz, a surgeon in the Prussian army, wrote a brilliant paper applying the principle to the sciences of physiology and chemistry. By the beginning of the twentieth century, the scientific observations of Rubner, and then Atwater and Benedict, had demonstrated the validity of the law of the conservation of energy for the human metabolism.

According to the law of conservation of energy – as related to humans – the energy value of the food eaten (minus the energy lost in waste) must equal the sum of the heat energy leaving the body plus the physical work done by the body. An overwhelming number of scientists today agree that weight change in human beings is linked to their energy balance (or imbalance), and that **weight loss in humans is governed by the law of the conservation of energy**.

Your Total Energy Requirements

How much energy do you need to maintain your present weight? To answer this question you must understand that an adult's energy requirement consists of three parts: 1) Basal metabolic energy, 2) Activity energy, and 3) Thermic energy. As illustrated in the following figure, the total amount of energy we expend everyday is the sum of the basal energy and the energy expended in physical activity. Our energy source is the food we eat minus waste.

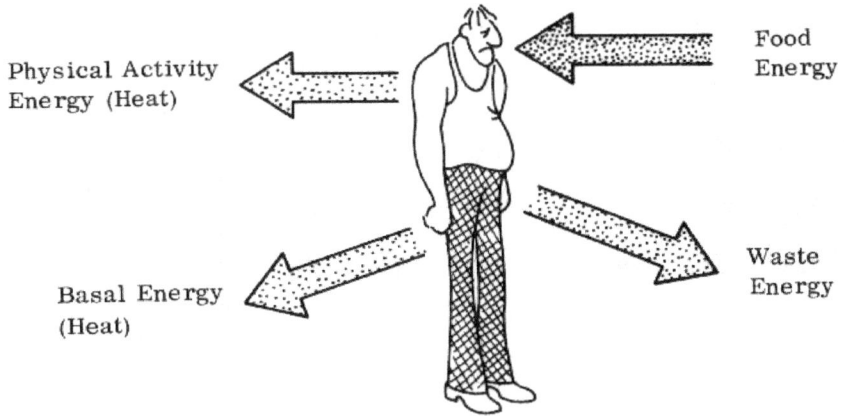

Physical Activity
Energy (Heat)

Food
Energy

Basal Energy
(Heat)

Waste
Energy

Basal Metabolic Energy

Basal metabolic energy is used to perform the body's involuntary basal processes, such as blood circulation, respiration, glandular activity, contraction of the intestines, body-temperature control, operation of the kidneys, etcetera. All of these functions consume energy. Scientists determine basal energy expenditure, also called basal metabolic rate (BMR), by a carefully controlled test in which measurements are made while a person who hasn't eaten in 14 hours lies quietly and completely relaxed in a comfortably warm room. Results from these tests show that basal metabolic energy is dependent on gender, age, weight and height, and that most people vary within plus and minus ten percent of what is considered normal.

When you reach your mid to late twenties, you slowly start to lose muscle and add fat as part of the natural aging process. But muscle is metabolically active tissue. This means your muscles use calories when they work, as well as when they repair and refuel. Fat, on the other hand, requires very few calories to exist. The conversion of muscle to fat as you age is the reason your basal metabolic rate decreases as you get older. (In general, women have lower basal metabolic rates than men because they generally have less muscle than men.)

Note that **a safe way to increase your basal metabolic rate is to convert fat to lean body tissue (muscle) by doing strengthening exercises**, such as those described later in this book

Activity Energy & Activity Levels

As soon as you begin to move about, the physical activity causes your energy output to increase significantly above your basal level. Many experiments have been performed to determine the energy used during various activities. Scientists express the results in terms of calories used per pound of body weight per unit of time. To compute your total daily energy requirement due to physical activity, therefore, would require that you keep a diary of the amount of time spent at each activity for an entire day; your total activity energy for the day would then be calculated by multiplying the amount of time spent at each activity by the caloric value per unit of time for each activity. This approach is fine in a science lab, but in the real world such a detailed determination is impractical.

To overcome this drawback, a number of years ago in an earlier publication this writer devised a more accessible measure of daily physical activity called the Activity-Level method. Essentially, to use the Activity-Level method, you make a judgment as to how active you are. Admittedly, this is the least quantitative topic in this book. Nevertheless, it is the most workable in practical, daily living situations. The two most common activity levels are covered in this text:

1) **Relatively Inactive During and after Work**: This is self-explanatory. It applies to individuals who sit at a desk most of the day and engage in no after-hours exercise.

2) **Moderately Active During or After Work**: To qualify for this category, you would have to either have a physically strenuous job (such as a construction worker, postal worker delivering mail on foot, etcetera), or engage in some form of regular exercise everyday after work (e.g., taking a brisk three-mile walk, working out in a gym, and so forth).

Once you settle on your Activity Level, you are ready to use the Weight Loss Prediction and Weight Maintenance Calorie tables in the sections that follow.

You Generate Heat When You Eat

In a classic experiment in calorimetry (heat energy measurement), the famous French scientist Lavoisier discovered that the ingestion of food caused an increase in the heat produced by the body. This heat increase is due to the energy required to chew and digest the food and to eliminate the waste. Nutritionists labeled this process the thermic effect of food or specific dynamic action. Note that thermic effect energy was taken into account in deriving the weight control equations used to produce the tables in this book.

Yet another factor that influences the amount of energy expended by the body is the ambient or environmental temperature. At low temperatures more heat is lost, but in temperate climates where people are well-clothed and houses are well-heated the effect of ambient temperature is negligible.

The Weight Control Program

You probably have tried many of the popular diets. I think you will agree that a major shortcoming of these popular quick-weight loss diets is that they lack quantitative information. In addition, many of these fads are neither medically nor scientifically sound. The Weight Control program is different!

How? First, it is the most logical and scientifically reliable weight-loss diet you will ever use. (You will be shown what to do and told why.) Next, the diet is based on the latest science. (You will develop an understanding that will allow you to choose among diet options. You will know numerically what is possible, what will happen and when.) Finally, the Weight Loss Program in this book is based on unassailable nutritional practices – no fads here. In short, you will be shown how to construct your own personalized weight loss program as follows:

1) Determine your activity level.

2) Set your weight loss goal and the rate at which you want to lose weight.

3) Determine your diet options from the Weight Loss Prediction Tables and choose your caloric intake and duration of your diet.

4) Analyze your eating habits and decide how to spread your calories, first among the days of the week, and then over the meals of the day.

5) Translate the calorie values into meal types and then actual food portions using a weight loss worksheet.

All of these points and more are covered later in this chapter. But before you start to plan your program, you need to understand some fundamental concepts.

When Does Weight Change Occur?

According to the conservation of energy principle, when the energy value of the food consumed minus waste, equals the sum of the basal energy and the energy expended during physical activity, the human body is said to be in energy equilibrium. In this case, that is **when the food energy taken in equals the total energy expended, weight is neither gained nor lost.** When there is an energy imbalance, however, weight is either gained or lost. In general, we can state:

- WEIGHT GAIN occurs when your food energy intake is greater than the total energy you expend. In this case your body stores the extra energy as fat.

- **WEIGHT LOSS** occurs when your food energy intake is less than the total energy you expend. In this case your body converts stored fat (and in some cases muscle) into energy.

The measure of energy, whether in the form of food, physical activity, or heat, is the (or the kilojoule or kilocalorie (hereafter simply called the kcal). As mentioned previously, weight loss occurs when you eat fewer calories than the calories you use in daily living. This difference in calories is referred to as the calorie deficit. How much weight you lose depends on the magnitude of the calorie deficit. In technical terms, **the calorie deficit, or calorie difference, is the driving force for weight change**. (Techies will appreciate that the calorie deficit which is the driving force for weight change is somewhat analogous to a voltage difference which is the driving force for the flow of electricity, and to a temperature difference which is the driving force for the flow of heat.)

What About Counting Carbs?

Every so often a low carbohydrate fad diet becomes popular and its adherents start monitoring the number of carbohydrate grams they consume. You will notice that no special mention of carbohydrates was made in the preceding section concerning weight change. This is because eating too many calories will result in weight gain, whether the calories are from protein, fat, or carbohydrate. In theory it does not matter what foods the calories are from.

Because carbohydrates contain 4 kcal per gram, if you restrict carbohydrates you are indirectly reducing the number of calories you eat, and you will lose weight. But why count carbs when it's calories that are causing the weight loss? In fact, researchers have shown that whether you are trying to lose weight or just maintain your weight, it's calories that count. In theory it does not matter what foods the calories are from – **to lose weight you have to eat fewer calories than you burn.**

Weight Loss Diets

Sure you want to lose weight but what diet should you choose? Low carb, high protein, low fat? Atkins, Zone, South Beach, Pritikin, or Ornish? What about the grapefruit diet or Sugar Busters? And on and on. Each fad diet that comes along promises to be the true path to weight loss.

In reality you can lose weight on almost any diet. Many of the aforementioned diets don't even mention the word calorie, but when analyzed carefully it's clear that by restricting certain foods these diets are in fact limiting calories. Again, you lose weight when you eat fewer calories than your body burns. It doesn't matter whether the calories are from protein, carbohydrates or fat. Calories are calories.

Low-fat diets gained popularity in the 1990's. And you can lose weight on a low-fat diet provided you also lower your calorie intake. But in recent years, even the strictest fat-limiting advocates have to admit that not all fats are alike. Some fats are bad for you (saturated and trans fats), but others are actually healthy (polyunsaturated and monounsaturated fats) and should be included in any diet – even a weight-loss diet.

Anecdotal evidence and weight loss research indicates that early on you will probably lose weight faster on a low-carb diet. The reason is two-fold. First at the start of any diet there is usually considerable loss of water – and water loss is particularly high for low-carb diets. But the main reason is that when you exclude carbohydrate-rich foods, you have no choice but to eat more fats and protein. Because fats and protein are digested more slowly than carbohydrates, most people don't feel quite as hungry on a low-carb reducing diet. So they eat less – eat fewer calories overall – and lose weight. The problem with low-carb diets is that most are nutritionally unsound and difficult to stay with. So what to do?

What Makes a Good Diet?

Every good weight-loss diet must have the following three characteristics:

1) A good diet must provide you with an understanding of weight control as well as the knowledge you need to reduce your weight to the desired level.

2) A good diet must help you remain healthy while you are losing weight.

3) A good diet must lead you to a healthier way of eating and exercising that will help you, in the long term, keep off the weight you have lost.

The weight-loss diet that fits these constraints is the so-called "balanced diet; " i.e., a diet that is not only low calorie but also nutritionally balanced and complies with the nutritional guidelines set forth in Appendix A.

Simplified Weight Loss Math

As stated previously, weight loss occurs when your food energy intake is less than the total energy you expend. This difference in calories is referred to as the calorie deficit. How much weight you lose depends on the magnitude of your calorie deficit.

People on any weight-loss diet invariably want to know how much weight they will lose – and how fast. Simple metabolic calculations make a rough estimate possible. Physiologists have long known that to lose one pound requires a deficit of approximately 7700 kcal. Therefore, if a person's total calorie deficit over time is known, their weight loss over time can be calculated.

As will be evident later, a 50 year-old male office worker, who weighs 71 kg, expends about 2500 kilocalories in day-to-day living. (In other words, if this man eats about 2500 kcalories per day he will neither gain nor lose weight.) If he goes on a 1500 kcal reducing diet, his daily calorie deficit would be 2500 − 1500 = 1000 kcal. In one week his deficit would be 1000 kcal per day x 7 days = 7000 kcal, and he should lose 7000/7700, or slightly less than one kilo.

This computation technique, however, is somewhat crude. Primarily because it does not account for a very important scientific fact: **As you lose weight you actually need fewer calories to maintain your lower weight.** As a result, if your calorie intake remains constant over some period of time, your calorie deficit will decrease during your diet and the rate at which you lose weight will also decrease with time.

Weight Loss Prediction Tables

Fortunately, a more precise determination of the rate of weight loss is possible. Scientists have long known that **weight loss is a function of age, sex, height, weight, physical activity, caloric intake and the duration of the diet (or time on the diet)**. This writer related all these variables in a complex, scientifically based, energy-weight-control equation, published in the *American Journal of Clinical Nutrition*,, and subsequently published a set of 60 Weight Loss Prediction tables. In this edition of Weight Loss for Men you will find an abridged set of six Weight Loss Prediction tables (Tables 14 through 19).

Selecting the Correct Table

Your first task is to choose the correct Weight Loss Prediction Table. The six Weight Loss Prediction Tables are organized by age and two activity levels. To repeat, the two most common activity levels covered in this text are:

1) **Relatively Inactive During and after Work**: (Hereafter often just labeled Inactive.) This is self-explanatory. It applies to individuals who sit at a desk most of the day and engage in no after-hours exercise.

2) **Moderately Active During or After Work**: (Hereafter often just labeled Active.) To qualify for this category, you would have to either have a physically strenuous job (such as a construction worker, postal worker delivering mail on foot, etcetera), or engage in some form of regular exercise everyday after work (e.g., taking a brisk five kilometer walk, working out in a gym, and so forth).

Use Table 12 to find the Weight Loss Prediction Table that's right for you:

Age	Activity Level	Table No.
18 – 35	Relatively inactive	**14** (page 31)
18 – 35	Moderately active	**15** (page 32)
36 – 55	Relatively inactive	**16** (page 33)
36 – 55	Moderately active	**17** (page 34)
56 – 75	Relatively inactive	**18** (page 35)
56 - 75	Moderately active	**19** (page 36)

Table 12: Select Weight Loss Table

Example:: Consider a 28-year-old man, who weighs 90 kilograms, has essentially a sedentary job as a computer programmer and spends most of his free time in front of a TV set. How long will it take him to lose 20 kilos?

First he should choose Table 14 labeled "Weight Loss Prediction for Relatively Inactive Men, Ages 18 - 35 years." (For this example please refer to Table 13.) Then he would scan the far left of the table and locate his present weight of 90 kg; from this number he would run his finger horizontally (to the right) until it intersects the vertical column headed by the 20 kg weight loss he desires. The three numbers at the intersection are the time in days for him to lose weight, depending on the diet calories consumed. Specifically, to lose 20 kg our fictional male's kcalorie intake options are:
- 1200 kcal per day for 105 days.
- 1500 kcal per day for 129 days.
- 1800 kcal per day for 168 days.

Which alternative should he choose? Health professionals recommend a gradual weight loss of about one kg per week. In this case, that would mean his diet should last about twenty weeks, or 140 days, pointing to the 1500 or 1800 kcal diet options. In the end, it comes down to deciding between a relatively shorter term 1500 kcal diet or a longer duration somewhat higher 1800 kcal diet option. Better still would be for him to increase his activity level by taking a brisk 5 kilometer walk everyday, and qualifying for the moderately active category (Table 15) which would result in the following shorter-duration diet options:
- 1200 kcal per day for 90 days.
- 1500 kcal per day for 107 days.
- 1800 kcal per day for 132 days.

Weight Loss Prediction for Men
(Relatively Inactive - 18 to 35)

Present Weight	Diet (kcal)	Weight Loss (kg)							
		5	10	15	20	25	30	35	40
60 kg	1200	38							
	1500	51				Numbers in table			
	1800	80				indicate time in days			
70 kg	1200	31	66	103		to lose weight.			
	1500	40	85	136					
	1800	56	122	202					
80 kg	1200	27	56	87	122	159			
	1500	33	70	110	155	206			
	1800	44	93	149	214	294			
90 kg	1200	24	49	76	105	137	171	209	
	1500	29	60	93	129	170	215	266	
	1800	36	75	119	168	224	290		
100 kg	1200	21	44	68	93	120	149	181	215
	1500	25	52	81	112	145	181	222	267
	1800	31	64	100	139	183	232	288	353

Table 13: Portion of Table 14

Please note that the kcalorie allowance during a weight loss diet need not be the same for every day of the week. It is the average intake over the entire week that counts. For instance, if the man in the example selected a 1500 kcal diet (which totals 1500 x 7 = 10500 kcal for one week), and his eating pattern is such that he knows he will invariably eat more on weekends, he could plan for 1200 kcal on weekdays and 2250 on weekends. In effect, he would then be dieting on weekdays and eating "almost normally" on weekends. This eating pattern would amount to (1200 x 5) + (2250 x 2) = 10500 kcal per week, which would result in the same weight loss outcome as if he consumed 1500 kcal each and every day of the week.

Weight Loss Prediction for Men
(Relatively Inactive - 18 to 35)

Present Weight	Diet (kcal)	Weight Loss (kg)							
		5	10	15	20	25	30	35	40
60 kg	1200	38				Numbers in table indicate time in days to lose weight.			
	1500	51							
	1800	80							
70 kg	1200	31	66	103					
	1500	40	85	136					
	1800	56	122	202					
80 kg	1200	27	56	87	122	159			
	1500	33	70	110	155	206			
	1800	44	93	149	214	294			
90 kg	1200	24	49	76	105	137	171	209	
	1500	29	60	93	129	170	215	266	
	1800	36	75	119	168	224	290		
100 kg	1200	21	44	68	93	120	149	181	215
	1500	25	52	81	112	145	181	222	267
	1800	31	64	100	139	183	232	288	353
110 kg	1200	20	40	61	84	108	133	160	189
	1500	23	46	72	99	127	158	191	228
	1800	27	56	86	119	155	195	238	287
120 kg	1500	21	42	65	89	114	141	169	200
	1800	24	49	76	105	136	169	205	244
	2100	29	60	93	129	168	211	259	313
140 kg	1500	19	38	59	80	103	127	152	179
	1800	22	44	68	94	121	149	180	213
	2100	26	53	82	112	145	181	220	263

Table 14: Weight Loss - Inactive - 18 to 35

Weight Loss Prediction for Men
(Moderately Active - 18 to 35)

Present Weight	Diet (kcal)	Weight Loss (kg)							
		5	10	15	20	25	30	35	40
60 kg	1200	32							
	1500	41				Numbers in table			
	1800	58				indicate time in days			
70 kg	1200	27	56	88		to lose weight.			
	1500	33	70	111					
	1800	43	92	150					
80 kg	1200	23	48	75	104	136			
	1500	28	58	90	127	168			
	1800	34	72	115	164	222			
90 kg	1200	20	42	65	90	117	146	178	
	1500	24	49	77	107	140	176	218	
	1800	29	60	94	132	175	224	282	
100 kg	1200	18	38	58	80	103	128	154	183
	1500	21	43	67	93	120	150	183	220
	1800	25	51	80	111	145	183	226	275
110 kg	1200	17	34	52	72	92	114	37	162
	1500	19	39	60	82	106	131	159	189
	1800	22	45	70	96	125	156	190	228
120 kg	1500	17	35	54	74	95	117	141	167
	1800	19	40	62	85	110	136	165	196
	2100	23	47	72	100	130	162	198	238
140 kg	1500	16	32	49	67	86	106	127	149
	1800	18	36	56	76	98	121	146	172
	2100	20	42	64	88	114	141	171	204

Table 15: Weight Loss - Active - 18 to 35

Weight Loss Prediction for Men
(Relatively Inactive - 36 to 55)

Present Weight	Diet (kcal)	Weight Loss (kg)							
		5	10	15	20	25	30	35	40
60 kg	1200	43				Numbers in table indicate time in days to lose weight.			
	1500	61							
	1800	107							
70 kg	1200	35	74	116					
	1500	47	99	160					
	1800	69	153	260					
80 kg	1200	30	62	97	136	179			
	1500	38	80	126	179	240			
	1800	52	111	180	264				
90 kg	1200	26	54	84	116	152	190	233	
	1500	32	67	105	147	193	246	307	
	1800	42	88	139	198	267	351		
100 kg	1200	23	48	74	102	132	165	200	238
	1500	28	58	90	125	163	205	251	304
	1800	35	73	114	160	212	271	340	
110 kg	1200	21	43	67	92	118	146	176	208
	1500	25	51	79	109	141	176	214	256
	1800	30	63	98	135	177	223	275	334
120 kg	1500	22	46	71	97	126	155	188	222
	1800	27	55	85	118	153	190	232	278
	2100	33	68	107	149	195	246	305	
140 kg	1500	21	42	64	88	113	139	167	197
	1800	24	49	76	104	135	167	202	240
	2100	29	60	92	128	166	208	254	306

Table 16: Weight Loss - Inactive - 36 to 55

Weight Loss Prediction for Men
(Moderately Active - 36 to 55)

Present Weight	Diet (kcal)	Weight Loss (kg)							
		5	10	15	20	25	30	35	40
60 kg	1200	36							
	1500	47				Numbers in table			
	1800	71				indicate time in days			
70 kg	1200	29	62	97		to lose weight.			
	1500	37	79	126					
	1800	50	109	180					
80 kg	1200	25	52	82	114	149			
	1500	31	64	101	143	190			
	1800	39	83	133	191	263			
90 kg	1200	22	46	71	98	127	159	195	
	1500	26	54	85	118	155	197	244	
	1800	32	67	106	150	200	259	330	
100 kg	1200	20	41	63	86	111	138	168	200
	1500	23	47	73	102	132	166	203	244
	1800	27	57	89	124	163	207	257	315
110 kg	1200	18	37	56	77	99	123	148	175
	1500	20	42	65	89	116	144	174	208
	1800	24	49	77	106	138	173	212	256
120 kg	1500	19	38	58	80	103	127	153	182
	1800	21	44	68	93	120	150	182	217
	2100	25	52	80	111	145	182	224	270
140 kg	1500	17	35	53	73	93	115	137	162
	1800	19	39	61	83	107	132	160	189
	2100	22	46	71	97	126	157	191	228

Table 17: Weight Loss - Active - 36 to 55

Weight Loss Prediction for Men
(Relatively Inactive - 56 to 75)

Present Weight	Diet (kcal)	Weight Loss (kg)							
		5	10	15	20	25	30	35	40
60 kg	1200	48							
	1500	72				Numbers in table			
	1800	145				indicate time in days			
70 kg	1200	39	81	129		to lose weight.			
	1500	53	114	186					
	1800	84	191	336					
80 kg	1200	33	68	107	149	197			
	1500	42	89	142	203	275			
	1800	60	131	215	321				
90 kg	1200	28	59	91	127	165	208	256	
	1500	35	74	116	163	216	277	349	
	1800	47	100	160	231	315			
100 kg	1200	25	52	80	111	143	179	217	260
	1500	31	64	99	138	180	227	280	341
	1800	39	82	129	182	242	313		
110 kg	1200	23	47	72	99	127	157	190	225
	1500	27	56	87	119	155	193	236	283
	1800	33	69	109	115 1	199	251	312	
120 kg	1500	24	50	77	106	136	169	205	243
	1800	29	61	94	130	169	212	259	312
	2100	37	77	121	169	223	284	354	
140 kg	1500	22	45	70	95	122	151	182	215
	1800	26	54	83	114	148	184	223	266
	2100	32	66	103	143	187	235	289	350

Table 18: Weight Loss - Inactive - 56 to 75

Weight Loss Prediction for Men
(Moderately Active - 56 to 75)

Present Weight	Diet (kcal)	Weight Loss (kg)							
		5	10	15	20	25	30	35	40
60 kg	1200	39				Numbers in table indicate time in days to lose weight.			
	1500	54							
	1800	86							
70 kg	1200	32	67	106					
	1500	41	87	141					
	1800	58	126	213					
80 kg	1200	27	56	88	123	162			
	1500	33	70	111	158	211			
	1800	44	93	151	220	306			
90 kg	1200	24	49	76	105	137	172	211	
	1500	28	59	92	129	170	217	270	
	1800	35	74	118	168	225	294		
100 kg	1200	21	43	67	92	119	148	180	215
	1500	25	51	79	110	143	180	221	268
	1800	30	62	97	136	180	230	287	356
110 kg	1200	19	39	60	82	106	131	158	187
	1500	22	45	70	96	124	155	188	225
	1800	26	54	83	116	151	190	234	283
120 kg	1500	20	40	62	85	110	136	165	195
	1800	23	47	73	101	130	163	198	237
	2100	27	56	88	122	160	202	249	303
140 kg	1500	18	37	56	77	99	122	147	173
	1800	21	42	65	89	115	143	173	205
	2100	24	50	77	106	138	172	210	251

Table 19: Weight Loss - Active - 56 to 75

Your Weight Loss Will Decrease

It is well known that if your caloric intake on a weight-loss diet is constant, your rate of weight loss will decrease with time. In other words, as you lose weight it will get more difficult, or rather it will take longer to lose additional weight! This declining weight loss rate will be illustrated for a 47-year-old man, who is relatively inactive, and weighs 90 kilos. Referring to **Table 16**, (page 33) you will notice that at the start of his diet, when he weighed 90 kg, on a 1500 kcal diet it took him 67 days to lose the first 10 kg. But the subsequent 10 kg took (147-67), or80 days! Why does this happen?

To understand this phenomenon you have to jump ahead to Table 25, (page 57) the Weight Maintenance Calorie Table which lists how many calories you can eat to neither gain nor lose weight. From Table 25 we find that before he began his diet, he must have been consuming about 2851 kcalories per day to maintain his weight at 90 kilos. At the start of his 1500-kcal diet, therefore, his deficit was 2851 − 1500 = 1351 kcal per day, and he would have started losing weight at a rate of (1351 x 7/7700), or approximately 1.23 kilo per week. At the end of his diet, the same table shows that at 70 kg he would have to eat no more than 2449 kcal per day to neither gain nor lose weight. His deficit then would have been only 2449 − 1500 = 949 kcalories per day, and his weight lose rate would have dropped to (949 x 7/7700), or about 0.86 kilos per week.

The lesson is that **if you want to lose weight at a constant rate over time, you must eat slightly less (or exercise harder) as you lose weight.**

Weight Variations Due to Water

When there is a calorie deficit the resulting weight loss is variable in its composition. Fat, water and protein (muscle, bone mass, etcetera) are lost at different rates at different times in the diet. A relatively high percentage of this weight loss is likely to be water, particularly at the start of a diet. For an average person water accounts for about 70 percent of their total body weight. Muscle tissue is approximately 75 percent water, 20 percent protein and five percent mineral. Body fat contains roughly 50 percent water. Because water is a significant component of weight loss, it is essential to understand how the amount of water in your body varies.

First, **realize that your body weight fluctuates about one kilo daily – whether on a diet or not.** Your weight is lowest before your morning meal and highest in the evening before retiring . In addition, the quantity of water in your body also varies from day to day. Over a reasonable time period, however, it can be stated that the amount of fluid leaving your body will equal the amount entering your body by way of food and drink. The water balance of your body is then said to be in equilibrium.

At the start of a diet, there is usually a considerable loss of water, and since 500 milliliters of water weighs about one-half kilogram, this initial water loss will appear to be a weight loss. But this weight loss is not "real" because only a small quantity of body tissue has been lost. (Many theories have been proposed to explain this phenomenon but none have been scientifically confirmed.) Changes in body hydration, therefore, cause a higher weight loss during the first week or two of a diet than is shown in the Weight Loss Prediction tables. By the following week, however, the body's water balance will again readjust and the total weight loss should more closely follow the values in the tables.

The Dreaded Weight Loss Plateau

Many dieters complain that after losing some amount of weight, they get stuck; they reach a so-called "plateau," and stop losing weight – at least for some time period. If this happens to you, you may get discouraged and frustrated and wonder what you should do to break through and start losing weight again. Before we address solutions, let's examine the possible causes of a weight loss plateau.

First, you could actually still be losing weight but at such a such low a rate that your weight loss is masked by the natural daily fluctuations in your weight, and your perception is that you have reached a plateau. The low weight loss rate is no doubt due to the much lower calorie deficit associated with your new lower weight – as described in the previous section "Your Weight Loss Rate Will Decreases Over Time." Recall, as you lose weight it gets increasingly harder to lose additional weight. If this is the case, the solution is to increase your calorie deficit by either reducing your caloric intake or increasing your activity level – or both. This done you should once more see a more detectable weight loss each week.

The most probable cause for a real weight loss plateau, however, is that over time you have become careless, either eating slightly more and/or exercising less. Yet another cause could be temporary water retention as discussed in the preceding section. More than likely it is a combination of all of these factors that makes you believe you have stopped losing weight.

If you encounter a weight loss plateau, the first thing to do is sit back and analyze your eating and exercise patterns. Keep a diet diary, honestly listing everything you eat and the associated calories. (Most people underestimate their caloric intake by at least 15 percent.) Add the calories consumed for a week and divide by seven to compute an average daily caloric intake. Then enter the Weight Maintenance Calorie table at your current weight and activity level and determine your maintenance calories. Next, calculate your all-important daily caloric deficit (maintenance calories minus your daily caloric intake). Then make an estimate of your expected weekly weight loss by multiplying your daily caloric deficit by seven and dividing the result by 7700.

Weight Loss Maxims

Once the parameters involved in weight loss are related in a mathematical equation, it is possible to state some principles or maxims. (It is also possible to deduce most of the following truisms by examining the Weight Loss Prediction tables.)

1) Given two people the same age, gender and activity level, and on the same reducing diet, **the heavier person will lose weight faster than the thinner person.** For instance, according to **Table 14** (page 31), on 1500 kcalories, it would take a 25-year old, 70 kg inactive male 85 days to lose 10 kilos; whereas the same table indicates a 90-kg man would only take 60 days to lose 10 kilos.

2) Given two people the same age, gender and activity level, and on the same reducing diet (i.e., consuming the same number of calories), the **taller person will lose weight at a faster rate.** (This phenomenon is shown in the more extensive original weight loss tables but height is not part of the abridged tables in this eBook.)

3) Given a male and female, the same age, weight, activity level and on the same reducing diet, **the man will lose weight faster than the woman.** This is because women most often have less muscle mass and, therefore, lower basal metabolic rates than men.

4) Given two individuals, the same gender, weight and activity level, **the younger person will lose weight faster than the older person.** The lesson is if you are overweight start on a weight loss diet now because it will only become **more difficult to lose weight as you get older.**

5) It follows that if your **caloric intake is constant over the years you will slowly gain weight as you age.** This is because you naturally lose muscle and your basal metabolic rate decreases as you advance in age, and most people tend not to be as active as they get older.

6) If your **caloric intake on a weight-loss diet is constant, your rate of weight loss will decrease with time.** Hence, to lose weight at a constant rate over time, you must eat slightly less (or exercise harder) as you lose weight.

Planning Weight Loss Eating Patterns

Using the nutrition and weight loss information presented to this point, you should be able to plan a reducing diet suited to your individual likes and lifestyle. This offers great flexibility, but requires that you take care and use the **Guidelines for Healthy Eating** (page 81) when choosing foods from all six-food groups.

After you determine your daily diet calorie allowance from the Weight Loss Prediction Tables, the next step is to decide on a weekly routine, i.e., how you will distribute your calories among the days of the week. As already mentioned your caloric allowance need not be the same for every day of the week. Next apportion your daily caloric allowance among the meals of the day according to your personal eating habits. The following approximate daily calorie distributions are suggestions only. (Feel free, however, to modify this calorie distribution to suit your particular eating routine and lifestyle.).

	1200	1500	1800
Breakfast	200	250	300
Lunch	250	350	400
Dinner	670	780	850
Snacks	80	150	250

Suggested Daily Calorie Distribution

Set Meals – Easier Calorie Control

Are you concerned about having to count calories? Whether on a reducing diet or trying to maintain your weight, allocating a specific number of calories for each meal makes it unnecessary to keep a running calorie tally for an entire day. Instead, you only need to monitor the number of calories eaten at each meal – and there are ways to keep even this to a minimum by utilizing a concept called "Set Meals" – a strategy not very different than the measured-food-to-eat systems used by diet plans such as Jenny Craig and NutriSystem. Except with the "Set Meals" system you control what you eat.

A Set Meal is a food serving where the ingredients vary - but is almost identical in calorie count and nutritional content day after day. Any meal during the day that is completely under your control is a Set Meal candidate.

For instance, suppose you prepare breakfast at home almost every day. Plan perhaps three set breakfasts. One might be based on cereal and fruit, another on eggs and toast, and so on. Variety is obtained by having more than one choice for a Set Meal, and by eating different kinds of cereal, or fruit, or egg preparations (scrambled, over easy, soft-boiled) – all within the same Set Meal. Once this is done, the number of calories in each of the Set Meal can be easily calculated. Then, try to plan set meals for lunch.

The more Set Meals you have in a day, the less calorie counting. If you have set meals for both breakfast and lunch, then you only have to monitor dinner calories.

Example: Devise a well-balanced, nutritious, weight-loss-eating plan for a 32-year-old man who wants to start on a 1500-kcal diet. He is married and works full-time as a nurse on the day shift.

First he has to distribute his 1500 kcal among the meals of the day. Based on his eating habits, as a first pass he decides to allocate approximately 275 kcal for his morning meal, 300 for his mid-day meal, 650 for his evening meal and 275 kcal for three snacks. (At this point, these calorie values are tentative and subject to change as his eating plan unfolds.)

Next, he has to establish his Set Meals, the meals he has control over, and also account for the foods he likes and dislikes. He certainly has control over his morning meal, and he has decided to bring a lunch to the hospital rather than eat in the cafeteria. So he also has control over what he eats for his mid-day meal. When he gets home from work, he and his wife prepare the evening meal together and sometimes they eat out.

In the morning he likes cereal with skim milk, or eggs and toast. For lunch he prefers things that are quick and easy to prepare like tuna fish, soup, cottage cheese, or cereal (if he hasn't already had cereal for his morning meal). He also enjoys a morning and afternoon snack. Now he is ready to layout his meal plan for every day of the week.

Using these facts as input, he establishes the weight loss eating plan broadly outlined in Table 20. Next, he calculates the number of kcalories in the foods comprising his Set Meals, i.e., his morning and afternoon meals and snacks. The details behind Table 20 are in a spreadsheet (not shown because of its size).

	Mon	Tues	Weds	Thurs	Fri	Sat	Sun
Morning Meal	Cereal (M)	Toast	Egg	Cereal (M)	Egg	Cereal (M)	Egg
Morning Snack	Fruit	Yogurt & Fruit	Yogurt & Fruit	Fruit	Yogurt & Fruit	Fruit	Yogurt & Fruit
Afternoon Meal	Soup	Cereal (S)	Cereal (S)	Tuna	Cereal (S)	Tuna	Cereal (S)
Afternoon Snack	Nuts& Seeds	Nuts & Seeds	Nuts & Seeds	Nuts& Seeds	Nuts & Seeds	Nuts& Seeds	Nuts & Seeds
kcalories	730	805	680	730	730	850	680

Table 20: Sample Weight Loss Eating Plan

For breakfast, "Cereal (M)" consists of a healthy cereal (such as Oat Meal, Wheatena, Farina, Shredded Wheat, Cheerios, Wheat Chex, Wheaties, and some Kashi cereals) with skim milk and topped with a half a banana or other fruit. "Cereal (Y)" substitutes non-fat yogurt for skim milk. In addition, ½cup of fruit juice are part of every breakfast.

For his mid-day meal, acceptable soups include tomato, vegetable, pea, actually any soup where a serving is 125 kcal or less. Any low-calorie salad dressing (about 25 kcal per tablespoon) can be used. Remember to use tuna packed in water rather than oil. Worth noting is that every effort was made to nutritionally balance the meals in a given day. For example, either milk, yogurt or cottage cheese are present every day.

Overall variety is achieved by having different brands of cereal, different kinds of fruit, several types of nuts and seeds, different kinds of soup, and eggs prepared in various ways. To make sure he is getting the proper amount of nutrients every day, for the evening meal he plans to have at least two other vegetable servings, a starch (potato or brown rice), and a small serving of fish, poultry, lean meat, or a plant protein. His evening snack (dessert) depends on the number of calories he has remaining after dinner. Dessert could be a small glass of skim milk and yes a cookie, or a low-calorie pudding, etc. Coffee or tea (with skim milk and an artificial sweetener if desired) can be served at any meal or as part of a snack.

From Table 20 we notice that his calorie total for breakfast, lunch and snacks is not the same for every day of the week. Because it is impractical to assign a different dinner calorie target for every day of the week, we average the daily totals for the morning and mid-day meals and snacks (as shown in the worksheet), and use the average value to calculate his allowable evening meal calories. Table 20 indicates that for his evening meal (and any evening snack) he is allowed a total of 756 kcalories (1500 kcalories minus the calories he has already eaten for his morning and mid-day meals and day-time snacks).

This evening meal kcalorie total should be relatively easy to stay within provided he eats well-balanced meals with portion sizes consistent with his 756 kcalorie limit. To understand what "reasonable" portion sizes should look like for a 756-kcalorie meal, at first he will probably have to count calories at dinner. After a few weeks of counting dinner calories, however, he should be able to judge what is and what is not an acceptable portion size for the different foods on his plate – and then proceed without actually counting calories.

Using this Set Meal technique, he only has to judge or estimate his evening meal calories to assure that he is close to his diet calorie allowance on a weekly basis. If you are uneasy about devising your own weight loss eating plan, either use the pre-planned diets in the next section, or seek the professional advice of a registered dietitian. Registered dietitians translate the science of nutrition into everyday information about food, and have the training to assist people with their individual diets and meal plans. Go online to find a registered dietitian in your area.

Finally, how should he manage the inevitable, i.e., when he has to attend a business luncheon, or an all-day business meeting, or he goes on a vacation? In other words, how should he handle those days when he just can't follow his weight loss eating plan? See **"Helpful Diet Strategies"** (page 47).

Pre-Planned Diets

Despite all the information that has been provided here, if you would rather not go through the trouble of planning a personal diet eating routine, use one of the pre-planned 1200, 1500, or 1800 kcalorie eating patterns shown in Tables 21 to 23. They are recommended because they adhere to the U.S. Department of Agriculture Dietary Guidelines and are nutritionally sound.

1200-kcalorie Diet

Morning Meal A	Morning Meal B	Morning Meal C
½ cup fruit or juice	½ cup fruit or juice	½ cup fruit or juice
30 g cereal	1 egg cooked w/o fat	30 g cereal
1 cup skim milk	1 slice dry toast	150 g fat-free yogurt
Coffee or tea	Coffee or tea	Coffee or tea
Mid-Day Meal A	**Mid-Day Meal B**	**Mid-Day Meal C**
1 cup no-fat cottage cheese	60 g lean meat	120 g fish
1 cup vegetables	1 cup vegetables	1 cup vegetables
Coffee or tea	1 slice bread	1 slice bread
	Coffee or tea	Coffee or tea
Evening Meal A	**Evening Meal B**	**Evening Meal C**
100 g lean meat	120 g fish	120 g chicken
Green salad + dressing	Green salad + dressing	Green salad + dressing
1 cup vegetables	1 cup vegetables	1 medium potato
1 slice bread	1 slice bread	1 cup fruit
1 cup fruit	1 cup fruit	Coffee or tea
Coffee or tea	Coffee or tea	
1110 kcal	**1120 kcal**	**1125 kcal**

Table 21: Menus for 1200 kcal Diet

Elective Calorie Budget: In addition to the above, 80 kcal may be used as desired for a snack - such as ½ cup non-fat ice cream, or for 15 g of peanut butter spread on a slice of bread, etc. **Note: 1 cup = 250 mL** (metric cup).

1500-kcalorie Diet

Morning Meal A	Morning Meal B	Morning Meal C
½ cup fruit or juice	½ cup fruit or juice	½ cup fruit or juice
30 g cereal	1 egg cooked w/o fat	30 g cereal
250 mL skim milk	2 slices dry toast	150 g fat-free yogurt
1 slice dry toast	Coffee or tea	1 slice dry toast
Coffee or tea		Coffee or tea
Mid-Day Meal A	**Mid-Day Meal B**	**Mid-Day Meal C**
1 cup no-fat cottage cheese	60 g lean meat	120 g fish
1 cup vegetables	1 cup vegetables	1 cup vegetables
1 slice bread	1 slice bread	1 slice bread
1 cup fruit	150 g fat-free yogurt	Coffee or tea
Coffee or tea	Coffee or tea	
Evening Meal A	**Evening Meal B**	**Evening Meal C**
110 g lean meat	150 g fish	150 g chicken
Green salad + dressing	Green salad + dressing	Green salad + dressing
1 cup vegetables	1 cup rice	1 medium potato
1 slice bread	1 cup vegetables	1 cup vegetables
1 cup fruit	1 cup fruit	1 cup fruit
Coffee or tea	Coffee or tea	Coffee or tea
1365 kcal	**1370 kcal**	**1340 kcal**

Table 24: Menus for 1500 kcal Diet

Elective Calorie Budget: In addition to the above, 140 kcalories may be used as desired for a snack - such as ¾cup low-fat ice cream, or for 15 g of peanut butter spread on a slice of bread, etc. **Note: 1 cup = 250 mL** (metric cup).

1800-kcalorie Diet

Morning Meal A	Morning Meal B	Morning Meal C
1 cup fruit or juice	1 cup fruit or juice	1 cup fruit or juice
30 g cereal	1 egg cooked w/o fat	30 g cereal
250 mL skim milk	1 slice dry toast	1 slice dry toast
1 slice dry toast	250 mL skim milk	250 g fat-free yogurt
Coffee or tea	Coffee or tea	Coffee or tea
Mid-Day Meal A	**Mid-Day Meal B**	**Mid-Day Meal C**
1 cup no-fat cottage cheese	120 g lean meat	150 g fish
1 cup vegetables	2 cups vegetables	2 cups vegetables
2 cups fruit	1 slice bread	2 slices bread
1 slice bread	2 cups fruit	2 cups fruit
Coffee or tea	Coffee or tea	Coffee or tea
Evening Meal A	**Evening Meal B**	**Evening Meal C**
150 g lean meat	180 g fish	180 g Chicken
Green salad + dressing	Green salad + dressing	Green salad + dressing
1 medium potato	2 cups rice	1 medium potato
2 cups vegetables	2 cups vegetables	2 cups vegetables
2 cups fruit	2 cups fruit	2 cups fruit
1 slice bread	1 slice bread	1 slice bread
250 mL skim milk	250 g fat-free yogurt	250 mL skim milk
1615 kcal	**1630 kcal**	**1600 kcal**

Table 23: Menus for 1800 kcal Diet

Elective Calorie Budget: In addition to the above, 185 kcalories may be used as desired for a snack - such as a cup of low-fat ice cream, or for 20 g of peanut butter spread on a slice of bread, etc. Note: **1 cup = 250 mL** (metric cup).

Notice that Tables 21 through 23 contain no recipes. For instance, the 1200 kcal Balanced Diet shown in Table 22 specifies ½ cup of vegetables, but does not identify the kind of vegetables and gives no advice regarding how the vegetables should be prepared. This is because Tables 21 to 23 are general diet guidelines around which more specific meals and recipes can be planned to suit individual preferences and taste. Admittedly, the menus

46

reflect typical American eating patterns but are easily modified to accommodate the tastes and traditions of people from other countries.

Again, if you are not sure you can devise your own weight loss eating plan, or the pre-planned diets in the next section are not to your liking, seek the professional help of a registered dietitian.

Notes for Pre-Planned Diets

The following notes apply to the 1200, 1500 and 1800 kcal diets shown in Tables 21 to 23

1) Cereal should be whole grain and preferably unsweetened. At the top of the list are Old-fashioned Oat Meal, Wheatena and Shredded Wheat. Among other reasonably healthy choices are Oatibix, Wheetabix, Wheaties some Kashi cereals and Farina.

2) Bread may be either plain or toasted whole wheat, whole rye or pumpernickel. If desired, bread may be sprayed with a zero-calorie butter substitute.

3) Meat should be lean cuts with all visible fat trimmed. Poultry should be limited to chicken or turkey breasts (white meat and skinless).

4) An unlimited amount of green salad may be eaten, but the salad dressing should contain no more than 10 mL of vegetable oil (olive, canola, sunflower, safflower etc).

5) Potato should be baked or boiled and (if desired) served with a dash of non-fat sour cream, or sprayed with a zero-calorie butter substitute. Where rice is specified, brown or wild rice is recommended.

6) Use freely as desired: clear unsweetened coffee, clear unsweetened tea, water (with a squeeze of lemon section if desired), seltzer water, and diet soda.

7) Use freely as desired: clear soups w/o fat, bouillon, and seasonings such as mustard, cinnamon, dill, herbs, red and black pepper, curry, vinegar, lemon juice and sections, and pickles.

Helpful Diet Strategies

Everyone needs strategies to help stay on the right-diet track. Here are a few time-tested dieting techniques that work. (All are explained in the sections that follow.)

1) Exchange equivalent foods for variety and prevent boredom.

2) To avoid "hidden calories," prepare simple foods cooked in an uncomplicated manner.

3) Get a good cookbook and a calorie reference.

4) Learn to estimate portion sizes.

5) Use Set Meals to make calorie control easy.
6) Handle occasional overeating by compensating.
7) Keep log of what you eat.
8) Use technology to monitor the calories you eat.
9) If it suits your lifestyle, follow a weekly rather a daily calorie allowance.
10) Handle special situations by temporarily going on weight maintenance.
11) Check your progress by graphing your weight loss.
Again all are discussed in some detail in the sections that follow. Choose the strategy (or strategies) that are right for you.

Exchanging Foods

To prevent a diet from becoming monotonous, after a few weeks try exchanging or substituting foods – a technique used by dieticians. Exchanging a food listed in a diet for another food with approximately equal caloric value and nutritional content is the foundation of a successful long-term diet. Substitution possibilities are almost endless but have to be done carefully.

The easiest substitutions are those within the same food group, such as exchanging one vegetable variety for another, or a glass of milk for a cup of yogurt. More sophisticated exchanges cross food groups, for instance replacing four ounces of lean meat with a tablespoon of peanut butter spread on a piece of whole wheat bread. Both foods are complete protein and both contain about 170 kcalories.

Simple is Better

When on a diet simple is better. Why? Because simple, uncomplicated meals will usually contain fewer "hidden calories" than more elaborate dishes. For example, straightforward broiled fish with micro-waved vegetables makes a nutritious, quick, low-calorie evening meal – with no "hidden calories." To add interest to foods without adding calories, season with spices and condiments.

Get Good Cookbook & Calorie Ref

Acquire a good low-calorie cookbook. Be sure the recipes cover morning meals, mid-day meals and evening meals, and all the recipes contain nutritional information, especially the number of kcalories per serving. In addition, **obtain a comprehensive food calorie guide** such as the excellent U.S. D. A. Home and Garden Bulletin No. 72: "Nutritive Value of Foods," which is online and can be downloaded at no cost.

Estimating Portion Sizes

Whatever kcalorie counting scheme you use, another dilemma for dieters is judging portion size. It makes no sense to worry about whether to apportion 300 or 350 kcalories per 100 grams for a cut of lean meat if you have no idea whether the portion you are planning to eat weighs 100 or 250 grams. You must learn to judge portion sizes with reasonable accuracy. The best way to do this is to start by weighing and measuring the food you eat. After about a week, your eye should be adjusted to what 100 grams of meat looks like, and you can then discontinue the weighing routine.

Incidentally, judging the weight of meat is one of the most important parts of many diets. As a guide, 100 grams of meat is about the size of a slice of bread 10 x 10 x ½ cm. And kcalorie tables always refer to meat that has been cooked and trimmed of visible fat and bone.

How to Handle Overeating

It's a fact of life that no matter how determined you are to abide by your daily calorie goal, life has a way of interfering. In real life, you probably will not be able to eat the same number of calories day after day. Maybe it's your social life that interferes. Maybe you have to attend a wedding reception. Maybe an unexpected occasion arises where you know you're going to go over your daily calorie allowance. What should you do?

The way to handle the inevitable overeating is by compensating. You compensate by estimating how far you have strayed from your weight-loss diet and then make amends at the next opportunity (usually the next meal or two) – by eating less.

For instance, let's say you have to attend a business luncheon. Further, assume the meal has been pre-ordered so you have no choice but to eat what's served. At some point toward the end of the meal, make a mental estimate of the number of kcalories you have eaten. Suppose, even though you tried to be careful, your estimate is about 850 kcalories. If your normal Set Lunch is 450 kcalories, you know you have over done it by approximately 400 kcalories. That night at your evening meal you decide to have water instead of wine, to forgo your evening snack and to take a half hour evening walk. By doing this, before the end of the day, you will have compensated for the extra 400 kcalories you ate at lunch.

Eating in Restaurants: To eat as few calories as possible, during your weight-loss diet adhere to the following restaurant guidelines. First, for an appetizer order fruit juice or melon. For your main course order broiled fish, poultry or a lean cut of meat cooked as plainly as possible (no butter, stuffing, gravy). Order steamed vegetables and maybe a baked potato.

Have your salad with the dressing on the side. Finally, ask for fruit for dessert – or have just coffee or tea.

Keep a Log of What You Eat

Behavior research indicates that dieters who keep a record of what they eat generally have more successful outcomes. How should you go about this? Keep a food log. A sample Daily Food Log is shown in Table 24 with one of the two days filled in. The dieter's goal was 1200 kcalories. The actual total for the day was 1240 kcalories. Not bad!

You can keep your daily food log in a small notebook, a laptop, a Smart Phone a handheld organizer, whatever works best for you. As shown, you should record the date, meal, food eaten, amount, calorie estimate, total calories for the day and any comments. To approximate the weight of a portion or serving use either a small scale or visually estimate the weight by employing rules of thumb, such as 120 grams of meat or fish is about the size of a deck of cards, and one and 50 grams of cheese is similar in size to a pair of dice. Once you know the weight, use either **Table 32** (page 89), "Calorie Rank (per 100 grams) of Common Foods," or a more comprehensive calorie reference to determine the calories in a particular portion.

Diet Tip: The secret to a healthy weight loss diet is to make every calorie count in terms of your nutritional needs.

Handling Special Situations

Suppose you are in the middle of your diet and you have to travel overseas for a few weeks, or you have to leave on a planned three-week family vacation. In both circumstances you know you will never be able to resist the food and stay on your diet. What to do?

One solution is to go off your diet – temporarily. Essentially go on weight maintenance and try to at least return from your trip or vacation without having gained any weight. (Weight Maintenance is covered in the next chapter where you will learn how many calories you can eat to neither gain nor lose weight.) When you get back, you can pick up where you left off – back on your diet and resume your weight loss.

Plot (Graph) Your Weight Loss

Another technique to help you track your weight loss progress, is to graphically compare your actual weight loss to your expected weight loss from the Weight Loss Prediction table that applies to you. If you're computer savvy you can plot your weight loss on your computer using a graphical software package. Otherwise, just use ordinary graph paper. Either way proceed as follows.

Meal	Food	Amount	kcal
Monday 07/12 Morning Meal	Juice Cereal Skim milk Black coffee	125 mL 30 g 125 mL	55 110 40 0
Snack	Tea		0
Mid-Day Meal	Cottage cheese Broccoli Bread	225 g 50 g 1 slice	160 25 75
Snack	Tea & cracker		60
Evening Meal	Salmon Baked potato Salad + oil Mixed veggies Bread Apple Skim milk	125 g Medium 15 mL 50 g Medium 1 slice 250 mL	200 100 140 45 75 75 80
		Total	1240

Table 24 Sample Daily Food Log

First, from the Weight Loss Prediction Table appropriate for your gender, age, and activity level, choose your diet calorie level. Next, using the data in the table, plot your predicted weight loss versus time on the diet. Draw a solid line through the data points. This is your baseline against which you will compare your actual weight loss. Weigh in at the start of your diet. Then, once a week, weigh yourself first thing in the morning and plot the value. If your weight loss is less than the predicted values, most likely you are either 1) cheating (eating more than your diet calorie allowance), or you are not as active as you think, as the weight loss prediction table you are using requires – or both.

Can You Target Weight Loss?

As you gain weight, a host of factors, the most important of which are genetics, gender, and age, determine where on your body you will put down fat. Let's say you have a particular area that's collected a lot of fat and it's bothering you – maybe it's around your abdomen (belly fat), your thighs or under your chin. Is there anything you can do to eliminate or just reduce the amount of fat in a particular annoying area? **The short answer is no**, but read on.

Losing Belly Fat

The truth of the matter is that your body decides where to put fat on and where to remove it, a system that is largely determined by your genetics. Your body distributes fat based on tactics developed over the eons.

Fat is stored in your abdomen, hips or buttocks because it takes less energy to carry fat accumulated in your midsection than other areas of your body. Keep in mind fat storage is a survival strategy, so your body tends to maximize energy efficiency in the formation, storage and use of body fat. Then, from an anthropological viewpoint, the location of body fat has reproductive implications. In women, fat is stored in the hips, buttocks and breasts to create a more attractive body in order to attract a potential mate. Lastly, your body amasses fat where you have put down fat cells when you were young.

Getting rid of abdominal fat has, undoubtedly, as great a level of misunderstanding as any weight loss subject. The major fallacy is that you can get rid of abdominal fat by working your abdominal muscles. This is based on the incorrect belief that fat is eliminated from a part of your body if you engage the muscles underneath that layer of fat. No such luck.

Last On First Off

This **general weight-change rule (based on observation) is "last on first off."** Assume as you gained weight, the first place you noticed it was on your thighs, next your buttocks, then your face. As you lose weight, it generally will come off in the reverse order, first from your face, then your rear and finally your thighs. And there is not much you can do about that. The truth is there is no food, no exercise, no magic belt, and no pill that will cause your body to lose fat in one place rather than another.

For women, this means the last place you're likely to lose fat is on your hips and buttocks. You may have already observed this phenomenon if you've ever been on a diet, or if you've lost weight but couldn't seem to lose that last bit of "stubborn" body fat.

For men, abdominal fat is probably the last fat that will disappear from your body. In the most likely progression, first you will lose fat from your face and extremities, such as your arms and legs, then from your upper torso, your chest, upper thighs and buttocks, and finally the fat stored in your abdomen. And science has not devised a technique to alter this fat reduction pattern.

So if you are really serious about getting rid of that abdominal fat, you're going to have to take a whole-body approach – and get used to the idea that belly fat is likely to be the last fat to go. This isn't what you want to hear, but it's the truth. To reduce body fat, you need to start consuming fewer calories than you expend on a daily basis. In other words, you need a calorie deficit. In time, your body will start converting fat into useable energy, and by doing so, fat stores will begin to disappear all across your body. But fat won't just magically vanish from one targeted place.

If you follow a healthy weight-loss diet combined with aerobic exercise and strength training, you will lose weight and eventually that weight loss will eliminate or reduce your particular problem area. In summary, despite what you may have read, there is no diet regimen or exercise routine that can "target" a particular area of your body. Just be patient and as you lose weight that problem area will eventually disappear.

Words of Caution

A reducing diet is best supervised by a physician. This is especially true when a great deal of weight needs to be lost, or if you have an ailment or a history of medical problems. The Weight Loss Prediction tables cover a wide range of possibilities. And while the values in the tables are theoretically attainable, they are not necessarily recommended for everyone. In some cases the wide ranges were computed and included for completeness.

Most physicians recommend that weight loss should be limited to no more than one kilo per week, except for very large individuals, or if the total amount of weight to be lost is very small. In these cases, an acceptable weight loss rate may be as high as three one and half kilos per week. And many nutritionists feel that weight-loss diets should not have food intakes below 900 to 1200 kcalories. This is because it is difficult to obtain the proper amount of essential nutrients below these levels.

Don't Give Up!

Finally, realize that, in all likelihood, the road to your weight loss goal will not be an easy one. You didn't gain all that extra weight last week, did you? No, of course not. You probably accumulated the extra weight over the course of several years. No doubt it was a slow, gradual change that occurred because your daily caloric intake during that time exceeded your daily caloric expenditure by some small amount. The point is that small but permanent changes in your diet can put you back on track and create the permanent weight loss you desire.

Don't get frazzled if you have a few setbacks along the way. Many dieters think that if they have a weekend or even a week where they eat more than they should, they might as well give up. Not true. Many successful dieters have lots of bad days. But they don't expect to be perfect. When you hit a bump in the road, simply take a break, relax, and re-start your diet. Successful dieters know that losing weight is a journey – with good days and some bad days – all are expected as they proceed along the road toward their weight loss goal.

3. WEIGHT MAINTENANCE

Most diet books either ignore or glance over weight maintenance. So the dieter who has somehow lost weight is left without any post-dieting guidelines regarding how to maintain their new lower weight. The purpose of this chapter is to help you maintain your hard earned weight loss.

The Weight Maintenance Program

In this chapter you will be introduced to the information you need to understand to successfully maintain your new weight level. You will learn how to apply the following to establish your own personalized a weight maintenance plan:

1) Use the Weight Maintenance Calorie Tables, to determine how many calories per day you may eat without gaining or losing a significant amount of weight.

2) Analyze your eating habits and decide how you will spread your maintenance calories, first among the days of the week, and then over the meals of an individual day.

3) Translate the calorie values into meal types and then actual food portions using a weight maintenance worksheet.

Again, each of these points will be elaborated on later in this chapter.

Why Do People Regain Weight?

Within five years, more than 90 percent of all dieters regain every pound they have lost. Why? In most cases it's because **after losing weight most people eventually revert to their pre-diet eating and exercising habits**, and this inevitably leads to their regaining the weight they lost – and often more. The fact is the less you weigh, the less you need to eat to sustain your lower weight. The quantity of food energy required to maintain a particular weight is again a function of sex, age, height, weight and activity level, as is clearly shown in Weight Maintenance Calorie Tables that follow.

   Within five years, more than 90 percent of all dieters regain every pound they have lost. Why? In most instances it is because after losing weight most people eventually revert to their pre-diet eating and exercising habits, and this inevitably leads to their regaining the weight they lost – and often more. The fact is the less we weigh, the less we need to eat to sustain that lower weight. The quantity of food energy required to maintain a particular weight is again a function of sex, age, weight and activity level, as is clearly shown in Weight Maintenance Table 25 on page 57.

Example: Let's consider a 53-year-old relatively inactive man who weighed 90 kilos at the start of his reducing diet. After losing 20 kilos, he weighed 70 kilos. Determine his weight maintenance calories before and after he lost weight.

From Table 26 find that before he started his diet, when he weighed 90 kilos, his weight maintenance level was 2851 kcal, meaning he must have been eating about 2851 kcal of food per day. After his diet, the same table shows that in order to maintain his lower weight of 70 kilos he must restrict his food intake in the future to 2449 kcal per day. On average, then, to neither gain nor lose weight at 70 kilos he must consume about 402 kcal per day less than he did when he weighed 90 kilos.

This person could help his cause by engaging in some form of exercise everyday. For example, if he walked 45 minutes every day at moderate 5.5 kph pace (covering a distance of slightly more than 4 kilometers), he could eat an additional $(305 - 90) \times 45 / 60 = 161$ kcalories per day without gaining weight. (See **Table 33**, on page 102 "Calories for Different Activities," and the related example.)

Life-Long Struggle

A study, published in the Annals of Internal Medicine, that followed 4000 people for three decades suggests that in the long term, 90 percent of men and 70 percent of women will become overweight (with a BMI $\geq$ 25). Interestingly, half of the men and women in the study, who had made it well into adulthood without a weight problem, ultimately also became overweight and a third became obese (with a BMI $\geq$ 30). The point being that you can never become complacent. **You must continually watch your weight because we are all at risk of becoming overweight.**

When you reach your mid to late twenties, you slowly start to lose muscle and add fat as part of the natural aging process. But muscle is metabolically active tissue. This means your muscles use calories when they work, as well as when they repair and refuel. Fat, on the other hand, requires very few calories to exist. This is one of the reasons you need fewer calories to remain at the same weight as you get older.

In weight maintenance, it is the number of calories you eat over the long term that is important. As an illustration, the weight maintenance value of 2449 kcal per day for the 53-year-old man in the previous example amounts to about 894000 kcalories in a single year. Now realize that an annual error of only two percent of this total (that is roughly 17900 kcalories per year, or 49 kcalories per day) would result in a weight gain of slightly more than 2 kilos in one year, and the importance of knowing and adhering to your personal weight maintenance calorie value becomes apparent. In brief, **to control your weight it is the number of calories eaten over the long term that matters**.

Weight Maintenance kilocalories

Weight (kg)	Age: 18-35 years		Age: 36-55 years		Age: 56-75 years	
	Inactive	Active	Inactive	Active	Inactive	Active
54	2232	2419	2102	2289	2002	2188
56	2279	2473	2147	2341	2045	2239
58	2325	2526	2191	2392	2088	2288
60	2371	2579	2235	2443	2130	2338
62	2416	2631	2279	2493	2172	2387
64	2461	2683	2322	2543	2214	2435
66	2506	2734	2364	2593	2255	2483
68	2550	2785	2407	2642	2296	2531
70	2594	2836	2449	2691	2336	2579
75	2701	2961	2552	2812	2436	2696
80	2807	3084	2653	2930	2535	2811
85	2911	3205	2753	3047	2631	2925
90	3013	3324	2851	3163	2726	3038
95	3113	3442	2948	3277	2820	3149
100	3212	3558	3043	3389	2913	3259
105	3310	3673	3137	3501	3004	3367
110	3406	3787	3230	3611	3094	3475
115	3501	3899	3322	3720	3184	3582
120	3596	4011	3413	3829	3272	3687
125	3689	4121	3503	3829	3360	3792
130	3781	4231	3593	4042	3447	3896

Table 25: Weight Maintenance kcalories

Obviously, it would be impossible for the man in the example to eat exactly 2449 kcalories day after day . Errors are inevitable and experience has shown that when people err they do so on the high side. They consume more calories than their maintenance value, rarely less. To allow for occasional overeating or days when you can't get in some exercise, it is recommended that you plan to eat about seven percent below the kilocalorie values in the weight maintenance tables. For the man in the previous example, that would result in about 2278 kcal per day rather than the 2278 kcalories shown in the weight maintenance calorie table – leaving him room for an occasional calorie splurge, or a missed exercise session.

Planning Maintenance Eating

Weight maintenance begins once you are at your "best weight," or achieve a weight that feels right for you. Weight maintenance is in fact more difficult than being on a weight-loss diet. Why? Chiefly because maintenance requires a life-long commitment, a commitment to a new life style where you eat balanced, nutritious meals that are within your maintenance calorie allowance.

Any motivational speech made at this point isn't going to be much help five and ten years down the road – when I trust you will still be in maintenance mode. Understand that if you really want to keep off the weight you have lost you will have to practice a good deal of self-discipline for a long time. Even the well motivated, however, need a good plan to succeed. The following approach (which is very similar to that discussed in the preceding "Planning Weight Loss Eating Patterns") is recommended:

1) Use the portion of the Weight Maintenance kcalorie table that applies to you to determine your daily weight-maintenance calorie allowance.

2) Then decide on a weekly routine, i.e., how your calorie allowance is to be distributed among the days of the week. (As stated previously our caloric intake need not be the same for every day of the week.)

3) Next allocate the daily caloric allowance among the meals of the day according to your eating habits. Obviously, a detailed meal plan for every possible calorie level cannot be included here, but given the information that is covered in Appendix A: Nutrition, it should be possible to plan eating patterns you can live with for any weight maintenance calorie allowance. (See the example that follows immediately). Granted this will take some work but in the long run it will be time well spent.

Example: Devise a weight maintenance eating plan for a 28-year-old man who, after losing 10 kilos, weighs 64 kilos. He describes his activity level as moderately active. An engineering consultant, he works from a home office.

First, from Table 25, he finds his maintenance calorie level is approximately 2541 kcal per day.) To determine how many calories per day he should plan to consume, he deducts a safety factor of seven percent from 2541 to allow for occasional overeating (or under-exercising). The result is about 2360 kcal per day – the number of maintenance kcalories he plans to eat on most days. Then, he has to establish the meals he has control over (these will be his Set Meals), and also account for the foods he likes and dislikes. Because on most days he is home all day, he has control over every meal except the evening meal. (When his wife gets home from work, they prepare dinner together or sometimes go out to eat.)

In the morning, the man in this example likes cereal (with skim or soy milk) or eggs, and for his mid-day meal he prefers a tuna sandwich, soup or cereal (if he hasn't already had cereal for breakfast). He also wants to allow for a morning and afternoon snack. Now he is ready to layout his meal plan for every day of the week. The resulting maintenance eating plan is broadly outlined in Table 26

Next, he calculates the number of calories in the foods comprising his Set Meals, i.e., his morning and afternoon meals and snacks. The details behind Table 26 are again not shown here.

	Mon	**Tues**	**Weds**	**Thurs**	**Fri**	**Sat**	**Sun**
Morning Meal	Cereal (M)	Toast	Egg	Cereal (M)	Egg	Cereal (M)	Egg
Snack	Fruit	Yogurt & Fruit	Yogurt & Fruit	Fruit	Yogurt & Fruit	Fruit	Yogurt & Fruit
Mid-Day Meal	Soup	Cereal (S)	Cereal (S)	Tuna	Cereal (S)	Tuna	Cereal (S)
Snack	Nuts & Seeds	Nuts & Seeds	Nuts & Seeds	Nuts & Seeds	Nuts & Seeds	Nuts & Seeds	Nuts & Seeds
kcal	1175	955	1075	1100	1075	1100	1075

Table 26: Sample Maintenance Eating Plan

As shown in Table 27, Cereal (M) indicates a cereal mix with skim milk, and that four ounces of juice are included with every breakfast choice. Worth noting is that every effort was made to balance the meals in a given day.

To assure he is getting an adequate amount of nutrients every day, for dinner he always intends to have a large salad, at least two other vegetable servings, a starch (potato or brown rice), and a small serving of fish, poultry, lean meat, or a plant protein. His evening snack (dessert) frequently includes a glass of skim milk and yes a few cookies. (Nobody is perfect!)

Overall variety is achieved by having different brands of cereal, different kinds of fruit, several types of nuts and seeds, different soup, and eggs prepared in various ways. In addition, to introduce even more variety, every few months he will revisit his plan and make some adjustments to his Set Meals by adding and subtracting foods.

For his evening meal, his kcalorie allowance is his maintenance kcalories minus the kcalories he has already eaten for his morning meal, mid-day meal and snacks Note that his kcalorie total for these meals is not the same for every day of the week. This is not unexpected. Because it is unrealistic to assign a different dinner calorie target for every day of the week, he averages the daily totals for his morning meal, mid-day meal and snacks (as shown in the worksheet), and uses the average value to calculate his allowable kcalories for his evening meal. In this manner, he determines that he can eat 1000 kcalories for his evening meal. This calorie total should satisfy the appetite of most men and should be easy to stay within provided he eats well-balanced meals with "reasonable" portion sizes. To understand what "reasonable" portion sizes should look like for a 1000-kcalorie meal, at first he will probably have to count calories at dinner. After a few weeks of counting evening meal calories, however, he should be able to judge what is and what is not an acceptable portion size for the different foods on his plate – without actually counting calories.

Using the Set Meal technique, he only has to judge or estimate his evening meal calories to assure that he is close to his maintenance kcalories on a weekly basis. This plan should make it easier for him to control what he eats and maintain his new lower weight over the long haul. Once again, if you are not sure you can devise your own weight maintenance eating plan, seek the professional advice of a registered dietitian.

Mini Diets Maintain Weight Loss

Many people go through life maintaining their weight without thinking about how much they eat or exercise. When they occasionally eat a bigger meal, they seem to automatically eat less at the next meal or they exercise more, or they do both. If for some reason they expend more energy, they instinctively eat more. These people are able to maintain an almost constant weight without any effort. For most of us, however, weight control is more difficult, and we must be vigilant. For most of us weight control is a relentless life-long challenge.

When on a weight-loss diet, check and record your progress by weighing yourself at the same time two or three days per week. Once you are in weight maintenance mode, i.e., you have reached your desired weight level, weigh in about once a week. Small, natural weight fluctuations can be ignored, but action is called for if you experience a "noteworthy" increase in weight. What is a noteworthy weight gain? For a 60-kg person a 2 kg increase would be noteworthy; whereas for a 95-kg individual a 4 kg weight gain would be noteworthy. Both would signal a call to action. Incidentally, for most people, over a lifetime, noteworthy weight shifts are all but inevitable. Nevertheless, you should **consider a noteworthy weight change a warning that you may be losing control of your weight and that you need to intervene to head off a potentially significant weight gain**.

If you need to lose two or five kilos to get back to your best weight, go on a short-term mini diet. Revisit the Weight Loss Prediction tables and determine the calorie level needed to lose about one kilo per week. For example, a 40-year-old moderately active 60-kg female on a 1200-kcal diet, should be able to lose two kilos in approximately 18 days, and a 40-year-old moderately active 100 kilo male on an 1800 kcal diet should be able to lose 5 kilos in approximately 24 days.

Once back to your best weight, revisit and analyze your weight maintenance eating and exercise routines and make any adjustments needed to keep your weight on target. Furthermore, appreciate that in order to maintain a proper weight level you may have to go on a number of short-term mini diets over your lifetime to correct small weight maintenance calorie eating errors.

Keys to Life-Long Weight Control

As with most pursuits, the earlier in life you begin the better. But regardless of your age, the sooner you start a weight-control program the easier it will be and the more time you will have to reap the benefits. So start on the path to sure weight control now! Despite all the detailed information presented in this book the path to life-long weight control is actually deceptively simple, and can be reduced to five basic keys. Assuming you have had a medical checkup, the five basic keys to life-long weight control are:

Key 1: If you are in maintenance mode, know your maintenance calorie value, i.e., how many calories you can eat to neither gain nor lose weight. Periodically you might experience a noteworthy weight gain. If this happens immediately go on a mini-diet.

Key 2: Practice good nutrition by eating a variety of foods from each food group – all within your caloric allowance. (See Appendix A which follows immediately.)

Key 3: Summarize your nutritional needs, i.e., how much of each nutrient and micronutrient should you be getting – via food or supplements.

Key 4: Engage in some form of moderate strength training at least two non-consecutive days per week.

Key 5: Engage in some form of moderate aerobic exercise every single day of the year. That is right every day! (If need be, cut back your aerobic workout on the days you do your strength exercises.)

To repeat, make every effort to engage in some form of moderate aerobic exercise every single day of the year! And try to exercise at the same time every day. This will probably mean rearranging priorities and putting exercise close to the top of your list. Soon exercise will become a part of your daily routine and you will not feel right unless you have had your daily run, or daily walk, etcetera.

Sure, there will be some days when it may seem impossible to fit exercise into your hectic schedule. Everyone would like to be able to workout for an uninterrupted hour, but the good news is that studies have shown that workouts as short as 15 minutes can improve your health. So on those very hectic, crazy days, try to fit in several 15-minute workouts whenever you can. Do the best with the time you have. Any other occasional additional exercise such as a round of golf on the weekend, cross-country skiing, attending a yoga class, is fine, beneficial, but should be considered secondary to your daily aerobic workout.

Appendix A: NUTRITION

In the opinion of many researchers the makeup of the diet eaten by the majority of people in developed countries is the single most important factor, albeit not the only one, accounting for our high incidence of overweight, and of death from coronary heart disease and stroke. Healthy eating habits, the result of sensible nutritional practices, must be an integral part of any weight control program. In this chapter you will learn how to improve the "nutritional quality" of the food you eat, and, as expected, we will also point out foods that you should avoid, i.e., those foods that are loaded with "nutritionally-empty calories."

Food is far more than just an energy source. Foods are made up of seven basic constituents: carbohydrates, proteins, fats, vitamins, minerals, fiber and water. (Some nutritionists would add phytochemicals to this list – but more on this later.) For healthy bodies you need to eat the correct quantity and proportion of all these components. You need protein, carbohydrates and fats, for growth, repair and energy. You need vitamins and minerals, albeit in relatively small quantities, so they can perform their vital roles in the thousands of biochemical reactions in your body. Fiber, the broad name given to the things you eat that your body cannot digest, is needed to assist your digestive system.

Fortunately, supermarkets have all the foods you need - and in abundance. Yet most nutritionists agree that a great many Americans are not eating well enough to sustain good health. In general, the U.S. diet is too high in fat – with an average of 40 percent of calories from fat – contributing to atherosclerosis. Another culprit is sugar. As a nation U.S. citizens consume more than 100 pounds of sugar per year per person, totaling an unhealthy, nutritionally empty, 500 Calories per day. This large intake of sugar leads to obvious ills, such as obesity and tooth decay. Add to this the increased use of processed and convenience foods, the proliferation of nutritional misinformation and deceptive advertising, and it is clear that you must improve your understanding of nutrition in order to eat properly.

Before we begin let's define some terms. Nutrients and micronutrients are the components of foods that are essential to human life. Proteins, carbohydrates and fats are nutrients. Some nutritionists refer to proteins, carbohydrates and fats as "macronutrients," and call vitamins and minerals "micronutrients" because they are present in foods in much smaller amounts than macronutrients. More recently, a new grouping of naturally occurring plant-based chemicals, called phytochemicals, or phytonutrients by some nutritionists, have been identified as having many healthful qualities, but unlike traditional macronutrients and micronutrients, phytonutrients are not needed by humans to live; i.e., their absence will not necessarily result in metabolic problems, or a deficiency disease.

Proteins

Proteins are molecules of amino acids that are required for cell maintenance and repair, as well as for the regulation of a wide range of bodily functions. Humans need 22 amino acids in order to live. Our bodies can make 14 of the amino acids on their own, but eight of them, called the essential-amino acids, must be acquired from the foods we eat.

Some foods have all the amino acids needed to build other proteins. These are called complete proteins. Nearly every animal food, including dairy products, eggs, meat, poultry and fish are complete proteins because they contain all eight-essential amino acids. Soy is the only plant-based food that has all eight essential-amino acids.

Other plant-based protein sources lack one or more essential amino acids (i.e., amino acids that the body can't either create, or manufacture by modifying other amino acids.) These incomplete proteins are found in legumes, grains, nuts, and seeds. However, consuming combinations of foods that have incomplete proteins can provide the same complete protein end effect as animal protein.

For a complete-protein meal, simply eat any of the incomplete proteins with another but different incomplete protein, such as eating legumes with grains, or legumes with nuts or seeds, or grains with nuts or seeds. Examples of some healthy plant-protein combinations (that provide complete protein) are pasta and beans, rice and lentils, corn and beans, bean soup with whole-grain bread, split-pea soup with whole-grain bread, peanut butter on whole-grain bread, and tortillas with refried beans.

Around the world, millions of people don't get enough protein. Protein malnutrition can cause growth failure, loss of muscle mass, decreased immunity, weakening of the heart and respiratory system, and in some cases death. Whereas, in developed countries, getting the minimum daily requirement of protein is usually not a problem, because almost any reasonable diet will provide most of us with sufficient protein.

Adults need about 0.79 grams of protein for every kilogram of body weight per day to keep from slowly breaking down their own tissue. A case in point, an adult weighing 70 kg requires about (70 x 0.79), or 55 grams of protein per day.

How much protein is in food? A few examples: There are approximately 25 grams of protein per 100 grams of beef, poultry, fish, cheese or peanuts. Soybeans pack 35 grams of protein per 100 grams. Most other beans and lentils contain about 20 grams of protein per 100 grams of product. There are roughly 10 grams of protein in 100 grams of whole-grain cereal, and milk has about 3 grams of protein per 100 mL.

Understand that foods are rarely straight protein. Some high-protein foods, such as marbled beef and whole milk, also come with lots of unhealthy saturated fat. Therefore, when you eat meat, eat the leanest cuts, and when you consume dairy products, choose skim or low-fat varieties. On the other hand, beans, nuts, and whole grains offer protein with little saturated fat – but with lots of healthful fiber and micronutrients.

You Need Carbs

Carbohydrates provide your body with its basic fuel, the energy your cells need to survive. The staple of most diets around the world, carbohydrates provide essential vitamins and minerals, fiber, and numerous beneficial compounds (phytonutrients) that promote good health.

The simplest carbohydrate is glucose. Also called "blood sugar" and "dextrose," glucose flows in the bloodstream so that it is available to every cell in your body. Your body's cells absorb glucose and convert it into energy to drive the cell. Glucose is a simple sugar, meaning that it tastes sweet. Some other simple sugars are sucrose, also known as "white sugar," fructose, the main sugar in fruits, and lactose, the sugar found in milk. They all taste sweet, and most are digested and enter your bloodstream quickly. When you eat fruit or drink milk, however, the natural sugar comes with vitamins, minerals (as well as fiber when you eat fruit); whereas the simple sugars in candy, for instance, are nothing but nutritionally-empty calories.

Then there are the more complex carbohydrates. Most grains (wheat, corn, oats, rice) and foods like potatoes, pasta and plantains are complex carbohydrates. In general, but not always, complex carbohydrates are digested more slowly than simple carbohydrates, and take much longer to enter your bloodstream. Most of us have heard that eating complex carbohydrates is good, and eating sugar-loaded foods is a bad. The reason is that simple sugars require little digestion, and when you eat a sweet food, such as a candy bar, or drink a can of soda, your blood glucose level rises rapidly. In response, your pancreas secretes a large amount of insulin to keep your blood glucose levels from rising too high. The large insulin response in turn tends to cause your blood sugar to fall to levels that are too low. As a consequence, about three to five hours after consuming sweets you feel lethargic and hungry. Many people react to this by eating yet another sweet, which can start a rollercoaster ride of surging glucose and then insulin. None of this is experienced after eating most complex carbohydrates, or a balanced meal, because the digestion and absorption processes are much slower.

Glycemic Index

Thinking of carbohydrates as complex or simple, as good or bad, is outdated. More recently, a system has been devised to classify carbohydrates. The system, called the glycemic index (GI), measures the effect a carbohydrate has on your blood sugar – quantifying how rapidly and to what level your blood sugar rises after you eat a food containing carbohydrates, compared to a reference food (usually glucose or white bread). For instance, a candy bar, which is digested rapidly has a high GI and causes an almost immediate jump in your blood sugar; whereas, lentil soup is digested more slowly and has a low GI. The factors that influence a food's GI are:

1) Fiber prevents the rapid digestion of the carbohydrates in food and slows the discharge of sugar molecules into the blood stream. Higher fiber content results in a lower GI.

2) Coarsely-ground grains are digested more slowly and, therefore, have lower GI values than finely-ground grains.

3) Less-processed carbohydrates, such whole-grain foods where the fiber, bran and germ are intact, are digested more slowly than highly-processed carbohydrates. In general, therefore, less processing usually results in a lower GI.

4) Unripe fruits and vegetables contain less sugar and have a lower GI than ripe varieties.

5) The more acid or fat a food has, the slower its carbohydrates are digested and absorbed into the blood stream. More acid and fat in a food mean a lower GI.

These factors sometimes lead to unexpected results. For instance, some foods containing simple carbohydrates such as fruit have a lower GI than a complex carbohydrate like the potato.

The glycemic index uses a scale of 0 to 100, with foods that cause the most rapid rise in blood sugar having the highest values. In this book and many others, glucose is the arbitrary reference food, and is assigned a GI = 100. (For a given food, a GI less than 56 is considered low, a GI = 56 to 69 is medium, and a GI greater than 69 is high.) Note that foods that contain little or no carbohydrate (such as meat, fish, eggs, avocado, wine, beer and other alcoholic beverages) do not have GI values.

Glycemic Load - More Meaning

Some food scientists have come to recognize that a food's GI value alone does not provide enough information to judge how a particular food will affect your blood sugar. This is because the GI does not take into account how much carbohydrate is in a food serving, and your blood sugar level is influenced by both the quality of the carbohydrate (GI) and the quantity of carbohydrate you eat. With this in mind, researchers developed a new guideline called the glycemic load (GL) which takes into account both a food's GI and the quantity of carbohydrate the food contains. A food's GL is calculated by multiplying the food's GI by the number of carbohydrate grams in a serving. For a given food, a GL less 11 is considered low, a GL = 11 to

19 is medium, and a GL greater than 19 is high. Most people consume 60 to 180 GL units per day, with a total GL of about 100 for a typical diet.

Table 27, on the following page, presents GI and GL values for some common foods. Most of the data are from the on-line database of the University of Sidney (Australia). The difference between a food's GI and GL is illustrated by a simple example. Table 28 indicates watermelon has a GI = 72, quite high. In this case, however, GI alone is misleading because watermelon only has about six grams of carbohydrate per serving. (Watermelon is almost entirely water, with some fiber and a small quantity of carbohydrate.) So a typical serving of watermelon, has a GL = GI x (net carb grams) = 0.72 x 6 = 4.3, which is quite low. (Note in the calculation, watermelon's GI value has been converted from 72% to the decimal equivalent 0.72.) Some diet book authors claim a food's GI and in some cases GL are the most important guidelines to use when planning a weight-loss diet. But consider the following: Pears (not shown in Table 27) are forbidden by some diets because of a relatively high GI = 40. However, a medium size pear weighing about 115 grams has a GL = 4, quite low. Now consider a 115 gram serving of peanuts with a much lower GI = 14, and an even lower GL = 2. For people on a reducing diet, based only on Glycemic Index or Load, a snack of peanuts appears to be a better choice than a pear. A medium-size pear, however, contains only 70 Calories, while four ounces of peanuts are loaded with about 650 Calories! Pears and peanuts are both healthy foods, but the extra 580 Calories in peanuts are certainly not going to help you lose weight.

Food	Glycemic Index (%)	Serving Size	Net Carbs	Glycemic Load
Strawberries	40	1 cup (150 g)	3	1
Peanuts	14	3.5 oz. (100 g)	9	1
Peach	42	large (120 g)	8	3
Carrot	92	large (80 g)	4	4
Lentils	28	1 cup (150 g)	15	4
Orange	48	medium (120 g)	9	4
Watermelon	72	1 cup (120 g)	6	4
Apple	40	medium (138 g)	15	6
Ice Cream	65	1 scoop (50 g)	10	7
Bread (wheat)	73	slice (30 g)	11	8
Grapes	46	4 oz. (120 g)	18	8
Bread (white)	70	1 slice (30 g)	13	9
Corn (sweet)	59	1 ear (80 g)	16	9
Banana	50	large (120 g)	24	12
Oatmeal	58	1 cup (234 g)	21	12
Sweet potato	50	medium (150 g)	26	13
Spaghetti	45	6 oz. (180 g)	44	20
Potato (baked)	94	medium (150 g)	22	21
Rice (brown)	50	4.5 oz. (130 g)	48	24
Raisins	64	1 box (60 g)	43	28
Rice (white)	72	4.5 oz. (130 g)	42	30
Snickers candy	55	1 bar (113 g)	64	35
Glucose	100	(50 g)	50	50

Table 27: Glycemic Rank of Common Foods

The focus on a food's GI can lead to limiting healthful foods that may have a high GI by themselves, but when eaten in combination with other foods are not a problem. A nutritious baked potato may have a high GI, but when eaten as part of a complete meal is digested more slowly than its GI value would indicate. The main point is that if you use GI or GL values as the sole factor when selecting your food, you could be eliminating very healthy foods, and eating too many calories and often too much fat as well. It is important, therefore, to appreciate that a food's GI and GL numbers only allow you to evaluate how a food's carbohydrate content affects your blood sugar level. Because our body performs better when our blood sugar remains relatively constant, we should be aware of a food's GL rank and consider it when planning our eating pattern. But there are other important factors that must also be taken into account, such as getting the micronutrients we need from a variety of foods, including carbohydrates, and staying within our caloric allowance.

In summary, **carbohydrates are neither all good nor all bad.** Remember good carbohydrates provide needed micronutrients. You should try to get the bulk of your calories from the good carbohydrates, i.e., from fruits, from vegetables and from whole grains such as whole-grain cereal, whole-wheat bread, whole-grain pasta, whole-old-fashioned oats, brown rice, bulgur, millet, and hulled barley.

Cholesterol and Triglyceride Levels

Atherosclerosis has been linked to both blood cholesterol and triglyceride levels. Both fatty substances are found in the plaque on the walls of clogged arteries. There are two types of cholesterol: high-density cholesterol (HDL), the "good" cholesterol, and low-density cholesterol (LDL), the "bad" cholesterol. You should have your cholesterol and triglyceride levels measured during a regular medical checkup and should know and understand the readings. At this writing, the desirable readings for otherwise healthy individuals are as follows:

- **Total cholesterol: less than 200 mg/dl.**
- **HDL cholesterol: greater than 40 mg/dl.**
- **LDL cholesterol: less than 130 mg/dl.**
- **Triglycerides: less than 150 mg/dl.**

For people who have coronary-artery disease, most cardiologists insist that the total cholesterol level be less than 160 mg/dl and the even more important LDL cholesterol be less than 100 mg/dl. Lately, cardiologists have been urging patients with coronary-artery disease to reduce their LDL even further to below 70 mg/dl.

Often, cholesterol and triglyceride levels can be reduced by adhering to the eating recommendations summarized at the end of the section that immediately follows, called "Fats in Foods." But where a low-fat diet alone does not work, people with high cholesterol and or high triglyceride levels, may be prescribed cholesterol-lowering medication by their physician. For more info on this important topic, visit the American Heart Association.

The Skinny on Fat

Fats are found in vegetable oil, seeds and nuts, meat and fish, and dairy products, as well as in foods like potato chips and french fries (that are cooked in oil), cookies, cake, and so on. There are certain fats you absolutely need to survive (the essential-fatty acids), and others you would do well to drastically limit (saturated fats) or avoid altogether (trans fats). Chemically, all fatty acids contain carbon chains with hydrogen atoms bonded to the carbon, and as you will learn later, all fats have the highest calorie density – containing nine calories per gram.

Until recently, the best wisdom was to eat a low-fat, low-cholesterol diet. This advice is now largely out of date. The latest research seems to show that the total amount of fat in the diet may not be strongly linked with disease. **What appears to matter is the type of fat in your diet.**

Saturated Fats: When all carbon bonds of a fat molecule are filled with hydrogen, a fat is said to be saturated, i.e., saturated with hydrogen atoms. Most saturated fats are animal in origin and are solid at room temperature (good examples are butter and the fat in meats). Generally speaking, you should avoid or at least severely limit your intake of saturated fats because they can raise both your total and bad LDL blood cholesterol levels which increases your chances of getting heart disease.

When hydrogen atoms are missing along the carbon chain the fatty acids are called monounsaturated or polyunsaturated depending on their exact chemical structure.

Monounsaturated fats (also called omega-9 fatty acids) are liquid at room temperature and are known as oils. They are "good fats" and are derived from plant sources, such as vegetable oils, nuts, and seeds. In studies in which monounsaturated fats were eaten in place of carbohydrates, LDL blood cholesterol levels decreased and HDL cholesterol levels increased. Monounsaturated fats are found in high concentrations in canola, olive and peanut oils.

Polyunsaturated fats are also liquid oils at room temperature and in your refrigerator. They are "good fats" and are derived from plant sources, such as vegetable oils, nuts, and seeds. Again, research has demonstrated that when polyunsaturated fats were eaten in place of carbohydrates, LDL blood cholesterol levels decreased and HDL cholesterol levels increased. Polyunsaturated fats are found in high concentrations in sunflower, soybean and corn oils.

Essential-Fatty Acids are class of polyunsaturated fatty acids that our body cannot create. These fats must be obtained from the food you eat. Essential-fatty acids promote absorption of the fat-soluble vitamins A, D,

E, and K and are also thought to provide many disease-fighting benefits. Because essential-fatty acids are needed and our body cannot manufacture them, they must come from the food we eat. Essential-fatty acids fall into two groups: omega-3 and omega-6.

Omega-3 fatty acids are relatively hard to find. Foods high in omega-3 fatty acids are walnuts, tofu, flax seeds and oily fish (salmon, mackerel, sardines, trout and albacore tuna). Omega-3 fats are thought to be heart-protective. (The American Heart Association suggests that people with coronary-heart disease consult with their physician regarding the advisability of taking a fish-oil supplement.)

Omega-6 fatty acids, on the other hand, are more common, easier to find, and are in most oils including sunflower, soybean and corn oils.

Current thinking is that the consumption of omega-6 and omega-3 fatty acids should be in the ratio of 3:1, with about three omega-6 for one omega-3. Many Western diets, however, contain about 15:1, omega-6 to omega-3, which is not good for your health. Although you need omega-6, people generally eat too much of it and not enough omega-3 fat. The American Heart Association recommends that you eat fish (particularly fatty fish) two times a week, as a way to get a more appropriate quantity of omega-3 fatty acids in your diet.

Fat Type	Where found
Saturated	**Meat, poultry (especially the skin), dairy products, lard, coconut oil, palm oil, cocoa butter**
Trans Fats	**Fried foods, margarine, snack foods, commercially-baked cake and cookies, and fast foods**
Cholesterol	**Egg yokes, dairy products, organ meats, fatty and prime meats, poultry skin, shellfish (particularly shrimp)**
Polyunsaturated (Omega-3)	Mackerel, salmon, sardines, tuna, canola oil, walnuts, flaxseed, wheat germ
Polyunsaturated (Omega-6)	Corn oil, cottonseed oil, safflower oil, sunflower oil, soybean oil
Monounsaturated (Omega-9)	Canola oil, olive oil, safflower oil (hybrid), sunflower oil (hybrid)

Table 28: Fats in Foods

In summary, it is becoming increasingly clear that saturated and trans fats, increase the risk for certain diseases while monounsaturated and polyunsaturated fats, lower the risk . The key is not to eliminate fat from your diet but to substitute good fats for bad fats, and at the same time try to reduce the total amount of fat consumed because all fats are very high in calories. The current scientific thinking regarding fat consumption is as follows:

1) Try to limit the total fat you eat to no more than 30 percent of your caloric intake.

2) Do not consume foods containing partially-hydrogenated vegetable oil because they are high in trans fats. This includes commercially prepared baked goods, snack foods, and processed foods, including fast foods. To be on the safe-side, assume these food products contain trans fats unless labeled otherwise.

3) Limit saturated fats, i.e., any fat of animal origin, to 10 percent of your caloric intake. Have meat less often, and when serving meat use lean cuts and trim the fat. Eat fish and poultry (white meat, without the skin) more frequently. Use fat-free or low-fat-milk dairy products in place of whole-milk dairy products. (Coconut and palm oil should also be avoided because they are saturated fats.)

4) When consuming fat, choose foods containing monounsaturated fats like olive oil and canola oil, and foods rich in polyunsaturated omega-6 and omega-3 fatty acids.

5) Try to balance your intake essential fatty acids by eating more omega-3 fatty acids, found in walnuts, tofu, certain seeds and oily fish such as salmon, sardines and tuna.

Vitamins and Minerals

The following is a listing of vitamins and minerals complete with a brief discussion of their function in your body, what foods supply the particular micronutrient, and the Recommended Dietary Allowance (RDA) – which is a reference number developed by the United States Food and Drug Administration to help consumers determine how much of a specific micronutrient a food contains. Summaries of the RDAs for vitamins are shown in Table 29 (page 75) and minerals in Table 30 (page 78). Notice that RDAs are frequently gender and age dependent, and pregnant and nursing women most often have special micronutrient needs.

Because of the rapid expansion of scientific knowledge regarding the role of micronutrients in human health, the U.S. Food and Drug Administration, in partnership with Health Canada, periodically assesses and updates the Recommended Daily Values. The following contains the recommended RDAs as of April 2006 for the vitamins and minerals discussed.

Vitamin A is a collection of fat-soluble compounds that play an important role in vision, bone growth, reproduction, cell division, and help prevent or fight off infections. Vitamin A also promotes healthy surface linings of the eyes, respiratory, urinary, and intestinal tracts, and also helps maintain the integrity of skin and mucous membranes. Using the long-established International Unit (IU) measure for the recommended dietary allowance (RDA), adult men and women need 3,000 and 2,330 IU (as retinol) per day respectively. However, the new RDA measure for vitamin A is the microgram (mcg), which translates for men and women as 900 and 700 mcg per day. Foods rich in vitamin A are orange-colored vegetables such as carrots, sweet potatoes and pumpkin; dark-green-leafy vegetables like spinach, collards and romaine lettuce; and orange-colored fruits such as mango, cantaloupe and apricots; and red peppers and tomatoes. One medium-size carrot supplies approximately 270 percent of your RDA.

Vitamin D is fat-soluble. Briefly, vitamin D is important in assisting the absorption of calcium, in forming strong bones and teeth and preventing deficiency diseases such as rickets and osteomalacia. For most adults, an adequate intake of vitamin D is 200 to 600 IU (which is equivalent to 5 to 15 mcg per day). In addition, your body can make vitamin D after exposure to sunshine. Good food sources include salt-water fish such as herring, salmon, sardines and fish-liver oils, as well as fortified milk and cereals. Small quantities are also found in egg yokes, veal and beef. An 250 mL glass of fortified milk supplies about 25 percent of your daily needs.

Vitamin E is a fat-soluble vitamin that is a powerful antioxidant and acts to protect cells against the effects of free radicals, which are potentially damaging by-products of energy metabolism. Research is underway to determine if vitamin E, through its ability to limit the production of free radicals, might help prevent or delay the development of cardiovascular disease and some cancers. For adults, the RDA for vitamin E is 22.5 IU (as d-alpha-tocopherol) which is equal to 15 mcg per day. Foods rich in vitamin E are vegetable oils, nuts, seeds, milk fat, egg yolks, liver, dark-green-leafy vegetables, and whole-grain foods. Approximately 12 almonds provide 100 percent of your RDA for vitamin E.

Vitamin K is another fat-soluble vitamin, and is known as the clotting vitamin because without it blood would not clot. Some studies also indicate that it helps maintain strong bones in the elderly. Adequate intake of vitamin K for men is 120 mcg per day and for women 90 mcg per day. Good sources are dark-green-leafy vegetables, soybean, cottonseed, canola, and olive oil. People who eat these foods as part of a balanced diet should easily get enough vitamin K.

Vitamin	Ages			
	19-30	31-50	51-70	70+
A (mcg)	900	900	900	900
D (mcg)	5	5	10	15
E (mcg)	15	15	15	15
K (mcg)	120	120	120	120
C (mg)	90	90	90	90
B_1 (mg)	1.2	1.2	1.2	1.2
B_2 (mg)	1.3	1.3	1.3	1.3
B_3 (mg)	16	16	16	16
B_5 (mg)	5	5	5	5
B_6 (mg)	1.3	1.3	1.7	1.7
B_7 (mcg)	30	30	30	30
B_9 (mcg)	400	400	400	400
B_{12} (mcg)	2.4	2.4	2.4	2.4

Table 29: Vitamin RDA for Men

Values for vitamins D, K, B_5 and B_7 are "Adequate Intake (AI)" because RDAs not established. mcg = micrograms per day mg = milligrams per day.

Vitamin C is a water-soluble, antioxidant vitamin. It is important in forming collagen, a protein that gives structure to bones, cartilage, muscle, and blood vessels. Vitamin C also aids in the absorption of iron, and helps maintain capillaries, bones, and teeth. The RDA for vitamin C is 90 milligrams (mg) per day for men and 75 mg per day for women. Foods rich in vitamin C are citrus fruits and juices, kiwifruit, strawberries, cantaloupe, broccoli, peppers, tomatoes, cabbage potatoes, and dark-green-leafy vegetables. A 180 mL glass of orange juice supplies 100 percent of a man's RDA.

Vitamin B is actually a complex of different water-soluble vitamins that often exist in the same foods. They perform an important role in our metabolism, in maintaining muscle tone along our digestive tract and in the health of our nervous system, skin, hair, eyes, mouth, and liver. The B complex vitamins are: vitamin B_1 (thiamine), vitamin B_2 (riboflavin), vitamin B_3 (niacin), vitamin B_5 (pantothenic acid), vitamin B_6 (pyridoxine), vitamin B_7 (biotin), vitamin B_9 (folic acid), and vitamin B_{12} (cyanocobalamin). Many cereals are fortified with all the B vitamins. Depending on the brand, one serving of a fortified cereal provides from 25 to 100 percent of the RDA for all the B vitamins (except vitamin B_7 biotin).

Vitamin B_1 (thiamine) plays a vital role in the proper operation of your nervous system. Your body also needs B_1 to convert carbohydrates into sugar and then energy. The RDA for men is 1.2 mg per day and 1.1 mg per day for women. Vitamin B_1 is found in meat, wheat germ, whole-grains cereals and breads, in enriched cereals and breads, in beans, nuts and seeds, and in dark-green-leafy vegetables.

Vitamin B_2 (riboflavin) also has a crucial role in certain metabolic reactions, particularly the conversion of carbohydrates into energy. Riboflavin is also an important antioxidant. The RDA is 1.3 mg per day for men and 1.1 mg per day for women. The best sources of riboflavin are brewer's yeast, almonds, organ meats, whole grains, wheat germ, wild rice, mushrooms, soybeans, milk, yogurt, eggs, broccoli, and spinach. In addition, flour and cereals are often fortified with riboflavin.

Vitamin B_3 (niacin) helps clear toxic and harmful chemicals from your body. It also assists in the production of various hormones. Niacin improves your circulation and reduces blood cholesterol levels. The RDA is 16 mg per day for men and 14 mg per day for women. Foods containing significant amounts of niacin are liver, meat, poultry, fish, whole-grains and nuts.

Vitamin B_5 (pantothenic acid) is necessary for a variety of life-sustaining tasks such as generating energy from food, synthesizing essential fats, and the function of your adrenal glands. Adequate intake of vitamin B_5 for adults is 5 mg per day. Good sources include organ meats, eggs, fish and shellfish, poultry, soybeans, beans, dairy foods, avocado, and mushrooms.

Vitamin B_6 (pyridoxine) is needed for protein and red-blood cell metabolism. Your body also requires vitamin B_6 to make hemoglobin. For men and women up to 50 years old, the RDA is 1.3 mg per day. After 50, the RDA increases to 1.7 mg per day for men and 1.5 mg for women.

Vitamin B_6 is found in a wide variety of foods including fortified cereals, beans, meat, poultry, fish, and some fruits and vegetables.

Vitamin B_7 (biotin) functions as a coenzyme in the synthesis of fat, glycogen and amino acids. An adequate intake of biotin is 30 mcg per day. A varied diet should provide enough biotin for most people. Liver, yeast and egg yokes are particularly rich food sources. It is also found in smaller amounts in fruit, meat and cheese.

Vitamin B_9 (folate or folic acid) helps produce and maintain new cells which is particularly important during periods of rapid cell division and growth such as in infancy and during pregnancy. Folate is needed to make DNA and RNA, the building blocks of cells. It is also thought to prevent DNA changes that may lead to cancer. For most adults, the RDA of folate is 400 mcg per day. Of course, women who are expecting or nursing need more folate. Cooked dry beans and peas, peanuts, oranges, dark-green-leafy vegetables and green peas are folate-rich foods.

Vitamin B_{12} (cyanocobalamin) enables your body to manufacture healthy red-blood cells. It also assists in the transmission of electrical signals between nerve cells. The recommended dietary allowance is 2.4 mcg per day. Vitamin B_{12} is found in fortified cereals, meat, fish and poultry.

Calcium is a mineral with several important functions. Most of the calcium in your body is used to support the structure of your bones and teeth. A small amount of calcium is in your blood, muscle, and the fluid between your cells. Calcium is also needed for muscle contraction, blood vessel contraction and expansion, the secretion of hormones and enzymes, and sending messages through the nervous system. For most adults, adequate intake is 1000 mg per day. Foods rich in calcium are milk, yogurt, natural cheeses (such as cheddar, Swiss and mozzarella), canned fish with soft bones such as salmon and sardines, and dark-green-leafy vegetables. 250 mL of milk (whole or skim) contains 30 percent of your RDA.

Chromium is important in the metabolism of fats and carbohydrates and in controlling blood sugar levels. It is an activator of several enzymes needed to drive numerous chemical reactions necessary to life. For men up to 50 years old, an adequate intake of chromium is 35 and mcg per day. After 50, the suggested adequate intake drops to 30 mcg per day. Whole grains, ready-to-eat bran cereals, seafood, green beans, broccoli, prunes, nuts, peanut butter, and potatoes are rich in chromium. 120 mL cup of chopped broccoli provides about 35 percent of your chromium RDA.

Iodine is a basic component of the thyroid hormone that regulates your metabolic rate. Lack of iodine can cause a number of physical and mental abnormalities. RDA for adult men and women is 150 mcg per day. Iodized salt, sea food and plants grown in iodine-rich soil are good sources of iodine. 100 grams of cooked haddock contains about 125 mcg of iodine.

Mineral	Ages			
	19-30	31-50	51-70	70+
Calcium (mg)	1000	1000	1200	1200
Chromium (mcg)	35	35	30	30
Copper (mcg)	900	900	900	900
Fluoride (mg)	4	4	4	4
Iodine (mcg)	150	150	150	150
Iron (mg)	8	8	8	8
Magnesium (mg)	400	420	420	420
Manganese (mg)	2.3	2.3	2.3	2.3
Molybdenum (mcg)	45	45	45	45
Phosphorus (mg)	700	700	700	700
Potassium (mg)	4700	4700	4700	4700
Selenium (mcg)	55	55	55	55
Zinc (mg)	11	11	11	11

Table 30: Mineral RDA for Men

Values for calcium, chromium, fluoride & manganese are "Adequate Intake (AI)" rather than RDA. mcg = micrograms per day mg = milligrams per day

Iron is an important mineral that aids the transport of oxygen in your body and is also needed for the regulation of cell growth. An iron deficiency limits oxygen delivery to cells, resulting in fatigue and decreased immunity. The RDA for iron is 8 mg per day for men and 18 mg per day for pre-menopausal women. Foods rich in iron are shrimp, clams, mussels, oysters, sardines, lean meats (especially beef), organ meats, turkey (dark meat), spinach, cooked dry beans, peas, lentils, and whole-grain breads and cereals. 100 grams of beef liver has approximately 50 percent of your iron RDA, and fortified cereals can provide from 50 to 100 percent of your RDA.

Magnesium is needed for hundreds of biochemical reactions in your body. It helps maintain normal muscle and nerve function, keeps heart rhythm steady, supports a healthy immune system, and keeps bones strong. The RDA is 420 mg per day for men and 320 for women. Dark-green-leafy vegetables, fish, some beans and peas, nuts and seeds, and whole grains are good sources of magnesium. One-half metric cup of cooked spinach has 75 mg of magnesium.

Phosphorus in combination with calcium is necessary for the formation of bones and teeth. Phosphorus is also involved in the metabolism of fats, carbohydrates and proteins, and in the effective utilization of many of the B vitamins. The RDA for adults is 700 mg per day. Rich sources of phosphorus are dairy products, meat, and fish. Phosphorus is also present in most soft drinks. Generally, a diet that provides adequate amounts of calcium and protein also provides a sufficient amount of phosphorus.

Potassium is involved in proper nerve function, muscle control and blood pressure regulation. (People engaged in vigorous exercise may need more potassium to replace that lost during exercise.) Low potassium levels can cause muscle cramping and cardiovascular irregularities. Adequate intake for men and women is 4700 mg per day. Potassium-rich foods include baked white or sweet potatoes, cooked leafy greens, winter (orange) squash, bananas, oranges, dried fruits (such as apricots and prunes), and cooked dry beans and lentils. A medium-size baked potato contains about 600 mg of potassium.

Selenium is an essential trace element that assists enzymes involved in antioxidant protection and thyroid hormone metabolism. The RDA is 55 mcg per day for men and women. The most important sources in American diets are meats, fish and grains. 100 grams of cooked cod provide about 32 mcg of selenium.

Zinc is an essential mineral that stimulates the activity of approximately 100 enzymes that promote biochemical reactions in your body. Zinc supports a healthy immune system needed for wound healing, and helps maintain your sense of taste and smell. The RDA for zinc is 11 mg per day for men and 8 mg per day for women. Oysters contain more zinc per serving than any other food. Other good sources are red meat, poultry, beans, nuts, certain seafood, whole grains, dairy products and fortified breakfast cereals which can provide from 50 to 100 percent of your RDA.

Phytonutrients: From Plants

Phytonutrients are not vitamins or minerals. Rather they are the beneficial compounds that give fruits and vegetables their many colors. "Phyto" comes from the Greek word for "plant," and that is where phytonutrients are found – in plant foods such as fruits, vegetables, whole grains, dried beans, nuts and seeds. Unlike traditional macronutrients and micronutrients (protein, fat, vitamins and minerals), phytonutrients are not necessary for life; i.e., they are not required for normal metabolism and their absence will not result in a deficiency disease. Despite this, research is expanding as evidence grows that phytonutrients have many beneficial qualities such as assisting the function of the immune system, reducing inflammation, acting directly against viruses, and playing a crucial role in preventing or reducing the risk of a number of chronic ailments, including heart disease, diabetes and cancer.

One of the most important roles of phytonutrients is as an antioxidant. Free radicals, which are by-products of energy metabolism, can damage cells and are thought to contribute to the development of cardiovascular disease and cancer. When antioxidant molecules encounter free radicals they neutralize them – limiting the damage. Our body needs more antioxidants as we grow older, because our body's ability to repair itself diminishes with age. Antioxidants are also thought to help prevent cell damage by environmental carcinogens.

Scientists understanding of phytonutrients is still in its infancy. Despite this, about one thousand phytonutrients have been identified to date and with ever expanding research new compounds are continually being discovered and organized into classes. The best known phytonutrient classes are carotenoids and polyphenols.

Carotenoids are contained in the yellow, orange, and red pigment in fruits and vegetables, as well as in dark-green-leafy vegetables (where the usual yellow color is masked by the vegetable's green pigment)

Some of the phytonutrients within the carotenoids class are alpha-carotene (contained in carrots); beta-carotene (in broccoli, sweet potato, pumpkin and carrots); beta-cryptoxanthin (in citrus fruits, peaches and apricots); lutein (in leafy greens such as kale, spinach and turnip greens); lycopene (in tomatoes, tomato paste, guava, pink grapefruit and watermelon); and zeaxanthin (in green vegetables and citrus fruit).

Polyphenol compounds are natural components of a wide variety of plants. Foods rich in polyphenols include apples, red wine, red grapes, grape juice, strawberries, raspberries, blueberries, cranberries, onions, tea, and certain nuts. Polyphenols are further subdivided into flavonoids and nonflavonoids.

Some phytonutrients in the flavonoids subgroup are anthocyanins (in fruits); catechins (found in tea and red wine); flavanones (in citrus fruit) flavones (in most fruits and vegetables); flavonols (in most fruits, vegetables, tea and red wine); and isoflavones (in soybeans). The nonflavonoids subgroup contains ellagic acid (found in strawberries, blueberries and raspberries).

Guidelines for Healthy Eating

No single food can supply all the nutrients you need in the amounts you need. The most important factors in nutrition are variety, variety, variety! **Variety is the key to a nutritious diet**. As a means of setting strategies for food selection, the U.S. Department of Health and Human Services and the Department of Agriculture issue Dietary Guidelines every five years. MyPyramid was replaced with **MyPlate** (see figure below). The 2015 Dietary Guidelines recommend the following:

• **Make Half your Plate Fruits and Vegetables:** Eat red, orange, and dark-green vegetables, such as tomatoes, sweet potatoes, and broccoli. Eat fruit, vegetables, or unsalted nuts as snacks.

• **Switch to Skim or 1% Milk:** Both have the same amount of calcium and other essential nutrients as whole milk, but less fat and calories. If lactose intolerant, try calcium-fortified soy products as an alternative to dairy foods.

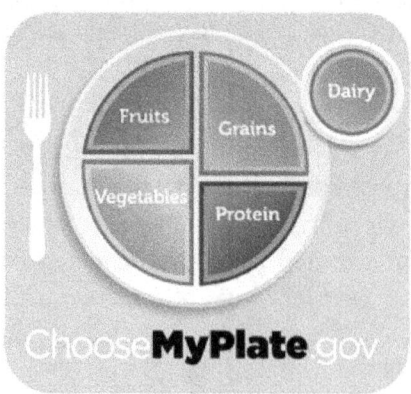

• **Make at least Half your Grains Whole:** Choose 100% wholegrain cereals, breads, crackers, rice, and pasta. Check the ingredients list on food packages to find whole-grain foods.

- **Vary your Protein Food choices:** Twice a week, make seafood the protein on your plate. Eat beans, a natural source of fiber and protein. Keep meat and poultry portions small & lean.
- **Choose Foods and Drinks with little or No Added Sugars:** Drink water instead of sugary drinks. Select fruit for dessert. Eat sugary desserts less often. Choose 100% fruit juice instead of fruit-flavored drinks.
- **Look Out for Salt (sodium) in Foods you Buy:** Compare sodium in foods like soup, bread, and frozen meals and choose the foods with lower numbers. Add spices or herbs to season food without adding salt.
- **Eat Fewer Foods that are High in Solid Fats:** Make major sources of saturated fats – such as cakes, cookies, ice cream, pizza, cheese, sausages, and hot dogs – occasional choices, not everyday foods. Select lean cuts of meats or poultry and fat-free or low-fat milk, yogurt, and cheese. Switch from solid fats to oils when preparing food.
- **To Maintain a Healthy Weight:** Basically enjoy your food, but eat less. Stay within your personal calorie limit. (Note that caloric needs will be covered in a later chapter.) Think before you eat: Is it worth the calories? Avoid oversized portions. Use a smaller plate, bowl, and glass. Stop eating when you are satisfied, not full.
- **Know your personal Daily Calorie Limit:** Keep that calorie number in mind when deciding what to eat. (Again, caloric needs will be covered in a later chapter.) Use a food log to keep track of how much you eat.
- **When Eating out Check posted Calorie Amounts:** Choose lower calorie menu options. Select dishes that include vegetables, fruits, and/or whole grains. Order a smaller portion or share when eating out. Cook more often at home, where you are in control of what's in your food.
- **If you Drink Alcoholic beverages, do so Sensibly:** Limit should be 1 drink a day for women or to 2 drinks a day for men.

Basic Food Groups

In this section we describe the various food groups, indicate what constitutes a serving size, and focus on the best foods within each group. (The foods in **bold font** are generally the most nutrient-dense foods – the best of the best.)

Fruit Group: Includes fresh, frozen, canned and dried fruits and fruit juices. A serving from the fruit group consists of approximately 130 grams of fresh, frozen or canned fruit, or 75 grams of dried fruit, or 250 mL of 100 percent fruit juice. This group can be divided further into citrus fruits, berries and grapes, and other fruits.

Citrus fruits: There are many excellent citrus choices including **oranges,**

grapefruit, lemons, limes, kiwifruit and kumquats. All are low calorie foods that contain a negligible amount of fat and cholesterol, are high in vitamin C, and most have significant amounts of vitamin A, potassium and dietary fiber.

Berries & grapes: Among the fruits in this grouping are **blackberries, blueberries, raspberries, strawberries, cranberries, gooseberries, purple grapes, black currents, raisins, and cherries**. Every fresh berry and grape is low calorie, with no fat or cholesterol, and all have small amounts of multiple micronutrients and a fair amount of dietary fiber. (Strawberries are also rich in vitamin C.) Some researchers claim that the blue and black-colored berries are packed with more disease-fighting antioxidants than any other fruit or vegetable. Of course, dark-red and purple grape contain the phytonutrient flavonol, the same antioxidant believed to give red wine its heart-protecting benefits.

Other fruits: This large subgroup includes a number of healthy foods such as **apples, apricots, bananas, cantaloupe, figs, mangos, papayas, peaches, pears, pineapples, plums, prunes and watermelon**. Again, most are low calorie, contain no fat or cholesterol, and are loaded with vitamins, minerals and phytonutrients. In addition, apples, apricots, figs, peaches, pears, pineapples, plums, prunes are good sources of dietary fiber. Cantaloupe is also high in vitamin C and watermelon contains the phytonutrient lycopene.

Vegetable Group: Includes fresh, frozen, dried and canned vegetables and vegetable juices. . In general, <u>one serving</u> from the vegetable group consists of about 130 grams of raw or cooked vegetables, or 250 mL of vegetable juice. This group can be broken down further into dark-green-leafy vegetables, orange-colored vegetables, starchy vegetables and other vegetables.

Dark-green-leafy vegetables: Every food in this category (which includes **bok choy, collard greens, kale, mustard greens, romaine lettuce, spinach, Swiss chard and turnip greens**) is low calorie with no fat or cholesterol, and is packed with micronutrients, especially vitamins A and C, calcium, iron, potassium and folate, as well as dietary fiber.

Orange-colored vegetables: The best in this subgroup are **carrots, orange-bell peppers, pumpkin, sweet potatoes, yams and winter squash**. All have negligible fat and cholesterol and are high in vitamin A, potassium and dietary fiber.

Starchy vegetables: This grouping overlaps somewhat with the orange-colored vegetable subgroup and the grains group. Among the foods included are **white potatoes, sweet potatoes, yams, yellow corn, and**

brown rice.   These vegetables are generally high in complex carbohydrates, B vitamins, potassium and dietary fiber.

Other vegetables: This extensive category contains **asparagus, broccoli, Brussels sprouts, cabbage, cauliflower, celery, cucumber, fennel, green beans, parsley, and summer squash**. The preceding are low calorie foods that contain a negligible amount of fat and cholesterol, and most have significant amounts of vitamins A and C, potassium, calcium, iron, other micronutrients and dietary fiber.   Also in this category are **eggplant, garlic, leeks, onions and mushrooms** which contain few calories, no cholesterol, and important amounts of potassium, calcium, iron and other micronutrients, as well as dietary fiber. **Red peppers and tomatoes** are low-calorie vegetables with no cholesterol that are loaded with vitamins A and C, iron and dietary fiber.   Tomatoes also contain the phytonutrient lycopene. **Avocado and olives** contain some beneficial monounsaturated and polyunsaturated fat, but no cholesterol. Avocados are relatively high in potassium and vitamin A, while olives have significant amounts of iron and calcium.

Grains Group: Includes all foods made from wheat, rice, oats, cornmeal and barley, such as bread, pasta, oatmeal, breakfast cereals and grits. One serving from the grains group consists of approximately 30 grams of bread (one thin slice), or 30 grams of ready-to-eat cereal, or 75 grams of cooked rice, pasta or cooked cereal. At least half of all grains you eat should be whole grains.

Grains are the seeds of varied grasses grown for food. The outermost layer of the grain is an inedible husk, called chaff. The next layer is the bran, a protective coating rich in fiber. When this layer is removed, the product is described as pearled or polished. Inside the bran is the endosperm (the starchy part of a grain) and the germ, the part highest in nutrients (e.g., wheat germ). Whole grains have all these components intact. Refined grains have the husk, bran, and germ removed. Many foods are a mixture of whole and refined grains. Check the ingredient list for the words "whole grain" or "whole wheat" to determine if a food is made from a whole grain. In the United States, to be labeled "whole grain" a food must contain more than 51 percent whole grain by weight.

Whole grains include: **barley, buckwheat, bulgur, corn, millet, oats, brown rice, rye, wheat and wild rice**. Some whole-grain foods are: **whole-wheat bread, whole-grain ready-to-eat cereal, whole-wheat crackers, oatmeal, popcorn, whole-wheat pasta**, and whole barley (in beef-barley soup). All grains are low in fat and contain no cholesterol.

Whole grains are good sources of complex carbohydrates and dietary fiber, as well as several B vitamins (thiamin, riboflavin, niacin, and folate), vitamin E, and minerals (iron, magnesium, and selenium).

Meats, Beans (and nuts) Group: One serving from this group consists of about 30 grams of lean meat, poultry, or fish, or one egg, or 20 grams of shelled seeds, or nuts (including peanut butter), or 30 grams of cooked dry beans. This group can be divided further into the subgroups meat and foul, fish, eggs, beans, and nuts and seeds.

Meat and Foul: **Skinless white-meat chicken and turkey** are relatively low calorie, low fat, low cholesterol foods that are powerful sources of high-quality protein, vitamin B_6, riboflavin, niacin, phosphorus and potassium. Most meats, even **lean meats**, are higher in fat and calories than chicken and turkey, but meats do provide high-quality protein and some important nutrients such as iron and B-vitamins.

Fish: Most fish are good choices including **cod, halibut, herring, mackerel, salmon, sardines, scallops, shrimp, snapper, trout and tuna.** Nearly all fish contain high levels of essential-fatty acids. (Oily cold-water fish such as wild salmon, sardines, herring, mackerel and tuna are high in omega-3 essential-fatty acid. Trout also has comparatively high omega-3 content.) All fish are relatively low-calorie foods and are good sources of the fat-soluble vitamins A and D. (Fish-liver oils have high levels of fat soluble vitamins, and have been used as dietary supplements for many years.) Nutritionally, seafood is better known for its dietary minerals than for its vitamins. This is because some minerals in fish, such as iodine and selenium, are not available at the same levels in most other non-marine foods. Fish are also a good source of iron and potassium.

There is, however, a downside to eating fish. Some fish are contaminated with mercury, PCBs, dioxins and other environmental pollutants. Mercury is a toxic heavy metal that can accumulate in certain fish species. Large predatory fish such as shark, swordfish, king mackerel and tilefish have the highest concentration of mercury and other environmental contaminates. Canned white albacore tuna, a commonly eaten fish, contains higher levels of mercury than canned light tuna . The U.S. Food and Drug Administration advises adults to eat no more than 180 grams of high-mercury fish per week.

PCBs are potential human carcinogens that find their way into fresh waters and oceans where they are absorbed by fish. A recent study reported that PCB levels in farmed salmon, especially those in from Europe, were about seven times higher than in wild salmon.

For further information about the safety of fish you catch locally, contact your local health department. If no advice is available, eat no more than 170 grams per week of fish caught from local waters and do not consume any other fish that week.

According to the University of Michigan Integrative Medicine Department, pregnant and nursing women, and young children, should avoid shark, swordfish, king mackerel and tilefish, and strictly limit the amount of other contaminated fish consumed.

Eggs: Current dietary guidelines and the latest research concerning egg consumption appear to be at odds. On the one hand, because a typical egg yoke contains saturated fat and 300 mg of cholesterol, the latest dietary guidelines recommend that egg yolks and whole eggs be used in moderation (up to one egg per day), but that egg whites and egg substitutes can be used freely since they contain no cholesterol and little or no fat.

On the other hand, others argue that if judged as a whole food and not simply as a source of cholesterol, positives such as the fact that eggs are low calorie, are loaded with high-quality protein, are a good source of vitamin E, etcetera, are apparent. Moreover, researchers at the Harvard Medical School studied egg consumption among 120,000 nurses and other health professionals with normal cholesterol levels and reported no link between eating eggs and heart disease or stroke.

Some medical researchers advise that, if one is at low risk (i.e., does not smoke, exercises regularly, eats a healthy diet and has no family history of heart disease or stroke) and chooses to begin eating eggs, they should have a blood test four to six weeks after they start eating eggs to determine the impact on their total and LDL cholesterol. Based on the test results, he and his doctor can decide – yes or no to him eating more eggs.

Beans: Among the foods in this important subgroup are **black beans, cannelloni beans, dried peas, fava beans, garbanzo beans, red kidney beans, lentils, lima beans, navy beans, and pinto beans**. All beans are inexpensive, low-fat, plant-protein-rich foods that are good sources of B vitamins, potassium, iron, dietary fiber and isoflavones (important phytonutrients).

Nuts and Seeds: This category consists of **almonds, cashews, hazelnuts, peanuts, pecans, pistachio nuts, walnuts, flaxseed, pumpkin seeds, sesame seeds, sunflower seeds**, and others. Because nuts and seeds contain significant amounts of essential-fatty acids, they are comparatively high-calorie foods. Most nuts and seeds have a good amount of dietary fiber, vitamin E, potassium, iron and folate. Almonds, cashews, peanuts, and pine nuts contain a significant quantity of plant protein and essential-fatty acids. Walnuts, flaxseed and pumpkin seeds are important sources of plant-based omega-3 fatty acids.

Soy: The soybean is the most widely grown legume. Healthful soy foods such as **tofu, soy nuts, soymilk, soybean oil, and soy protein** are made from soybeans. All contain a significant amount of plant-based complete protein and omega-3 fatty acid as well as vitamin E, potassium, iron and folate. Soy nuts are also high in dietary fiber.

Soybeans, tofu, and other soy-based foods are an excellent alternative to red meat. But there are some suspected dangers from too much soy. So do not to overdo it. The Harvard University School of Public Health recommends two to four servings of soy foods per week as a good goal. Furthermore, they caution adults not to take supplements that contain concentrated soy protein or soy extracts, such as isoflavones.

Milk Group: Includes liquid milk and all products and foods made from milk such yogurt and cheese. (Foods that have little or no calcium such as cream, butter and cream cheese are not in this group.) One serving from the milk group consists of 250 mL of milk or yogurt, or 40 grams of natural cheese, or 60 grams of processed cheese.

Milk, yogurt and natural cheeses are high in calcium and protein. **Milk** is also often fortified with vitamin D. In addition to calcium and protein, **yogurt** is a particularly wholesome food providing live active bacteria cultures which promote gastrointestinal health. Most choices in this group should be fat free or low fat.

Oils Group: Includes vegetable oils and foods such as **nuts, olives, oily fish, avocados**, mayonnaise, soft margarine and some salad dressings. You should limit the intake of saturated fats – that is any fat of animal origin.

The oils group overlaps somewhat with many of the others. Liquid oils, however, are unique to this group. **Corn oil, flaxseed oil, safflower oil, sesame oil, soybean oil and sunflower oil** are polyunsaturated; whereas, **canola oil, olive oil and peanut oil** are monounsaturated. All these oils are high in calories and essential-fatty acids. Essential-fatty acids promote absorption of the fat-soluble vitamins A, D, E, and K. Flaxseed, canola and soybean oil contain omega-3 fatty acids. (Note, when purchasing olive oil, choose an oil that is labeled "extra-virgin" or "virgin." Virgin olive oils are produced from the first pressing of the olives, are unrefined and as a result are more healthful.)

➡ Everyone should have a medical checkup before making major changes to their eating patterns. This is particularly important for anyone with medical problems and for women who are pregnant or breast- feeding, all of whom should consult a physician, nutritionist or registered dietician to determine the dietary pattern that is appropriate for them.

Vitamin/Mineral Supplements

Even though most adults can get all the vitamins and minerals they need by merely consuming a variety of nutritious foods (from the fruit group, the vegetable group, the grains group, the meat and beans group, the milk group, and the oils group), **many physicians recommend a daily multi-vitamin/mineral supplement as a kind of insurance policy**.

Be aware that some micronutrients, such as the fat-soluble vitamin A, can be harmful if taken in large quantities. To be safe your multi-vitamin/mineral supplement should contain no more than 100 percent of the recommended dietary allowance (RDA) for each vitamin or mineral. Generally, you don't need the high doses in multi-vitamin/mineral supplements labeled "therapeutic" or "extra-strength." There may be medical reasons for taking larger amounts of a vitamin or mineral than the RDA provides, but check with your doctor first. For example, a physician may advise a pregnant woman to take an iron supplement, and women who could become pregnant to take folic acid in addition to consuming folate-rich foods to reduce the risk of some serious birth defects. Adults over age 50 and vegetarians who do not eat animal foods may be advised to get their vitamin B_{12} from a supplement or from fortified foods. People with little exposure to sunlight may need a vitamin D supplement, and individuals who seldom eat dairy products or other rich sources of calcium may need to take a calcium supplement.

Dietary supplement choices include not only vitamins and minerals, but also herbal products and many other widely available substances. Herbal products, however, usually provide only small amounts of vitamins and minerals and their health value is currently being studied.

Become a Calorie Expert

In order to plan a diet you must be able to estimate the calorie value of foods as well as portion sizes. The Nutrition Facts label on food packages, listing nutrient content, makes it possible to calculate the number of calories in a serving if you know that there are roughly:

	Calories per gram
Carbohydrates	4
Protein	4
Alcohol	7
Fat	9

Example **Example** Determine the calories in a cup 250 mL of whole milk. The label on a container of whole milk indicates that a cup has 11 grams of carbohydrate, 8 grams of protein and 9 grams of fat. Therefore, the total calories in 250 mL of whole milk can be determined as follows:

11 gms carbs x 4 Cal per gm = 44 Cal
8 gms protein x 4 Cal per gm = 32 Cal
9 gms fat x 9 Cal per gm = 81 Cal
Total = 44+32+81 = <u>157 Calories</u>

A sense of the caloric value (per 100g) of some <u>basic foods</u> can be obtained from Table 31. The extremes of the chart are represented by water the lowest, at zero kcalories, and fat (lard) the highest at about 900 kcalories per 100 grams. Sugar (a pure carbohydrate) is near the middle of the ranking at 400 kcalories per 100g. Protein is also approximately 400 kcalories per 100g but there is no pure protein food to rank. (Note, most of the kcalorie values in Table 31 are the average of many varieties in a particular category.)

Table 31: Calorie Rank of Basic Foods

Water	0	Pasta	125
Coffee or Tea	4	Fish	145
Vegetables	20	Egg	163
Milk (fat free)	32	Poultry	188
Soft drink	42	Bread	248
Beer	44	Whiskey	249
Fruit	60	Meat	320
Milk (whole)	66	Cake	350
Potato	76	Sugar	400
Corn	87	Chocolate	530
Wine	88	Nuts	615
Rice	114	Vegetable oil	884
Beans	118	Lard	900

Table 32 is an expanded version of the previous table that includes the **kcal per 100 g** of some commonly encountered foods.

Water	0	Peas	71	Liverwurst	278
Coffee/Tea	4	Yogurt (whole)	73	Hamburger	286
Vinegar	9	Potato (boiled)	76	Tuna (in oil)	288
Lettuce	15	Clams (raw)	79	Raisins	290
Celery	16	Banana	85	Bologna	304
Asparagus	23	Corn	87	Wheat Flakes	310
Tomato	24	Wine	88	Cake (average)	350
Spinach	25	Lobster	93	Sirloin Steak	360
Watermelon	26	Lentils	106	Cheese	370
Lemon	27	Scallops	112	Ham (baked)	370
Broccoli	28	Rice	114	Oatmeal	375
Mushrooms	30	Beans	118	Sugar	400
Cantaloupe	30	Pasta	125	Pretzels	390
Milk (fat free)	32	Tuna (in water)	127	Crackers	400
Carrots	36	Olives (black)	129	Doughnut	410
Strawberries	37	Blue Fish (baked)	159	Fudge	410
Green Pepper	37	Egg (boiled)	163	Chocolate	530
Peach	38	Turkey (light)	176	Potato Chips	568
Grapefruit	40	Ice Cream	193	Peanut Butter	585
Cola Drink	42	Sardines	196	Almonds	598
Beer	44	Turkey (dark)	203	Bacon	611
Yogurt (no fat)	44	Pancakes	225	Walnuts	630
Orange	50	Bread (wheat)	243	Butter	716
Apple	56	Whisky-86 proof	249	Mayonnaise	718
Milk (whole)	66	Apple Pie	256	Margarine	720
Cherries	68	Bread (white)	270	Vegetable Oil	884
Grapes	68	Jam/Jelly	272	Lard (fat)	900

Table 32: Calorie Rank of Common Foods

If you appreciate that **all foods are some combination of water, carbohydrate, protein, fat and fiber**, this can lead to a better understanding of why a particular food has the caloric value
and rank shown in the table. For example, watermelon is almost entirely water, with some fiber (zero kcalories) and carbohydrate, with no protein or fat, and consequently has a very low kcalorie per 100 gram value. A grape is again mostly water with some fiber and carbohydrate and according to the chart has only 68 kcal per 100 grams, but a raisin (a dried grape) is almost entirely carbohydrate and fiber with little water and thus has a value of 290 kcal per 100 grams – closer to a pure carbohydrate.

When a food is not listed in the chart, common sense can often be used to estimate its calorie value; e.g., green beans are not listed, but judging from the ranking of similar foods a value of 20 kcal per 100 grams seems reasonable. Table 32 can also be thought of as a listing of the "calorie density" of foods. As an example, the table illustrates that one kilo of carrots contains about 360 kcal, or approximately the same number of kcalories as 100 grams of sirloin steak at 360 kcal. (Note that the numbers in the table are approximate kcalories per 100 grams of fluid or dry weight.) Moreover, Table 32 in combination with a small weighing scale makes a very useful diet aide - allowing the calorie value of many food portions to be estimated quite accurately. It is a simple mater to weigh a piece of meat or a pancake, or a slice of apple pie, and multiple the weight in grams by the kcalorie value per 100 grams (from Table 32) and divide by 100 to determine the total number of kcalories. Frequently, the preceding approach will result in more precise calorie values than those obtained from the numbers shown in an ordinary calorie table where the portion size is often ambiguously described.

Estimating Calories in a Meal

As discussed, you must be able to judge the caloric value of foods if you are going to successfully control your weight. Another useful technique in this regard is to use an engineering-like approach. The first thing an engineer does when performing most calculations is to "ball-park" the answer. You will often hear an engineer remark, "Should the diameter of that shaft (for example) be one inch or ten inches? What ball-park are we in?" Initially he or she does a relatively crude, quick, over-simplified calculation that yields a "ball-park" answer. Later, time and circumstances permitting, the engineer will go back and do a more thorough analysis, considering all the subtleties of the problem. It is recommended that you approach calorie counting in much the same manner.

90

For example, you're having a meal with friends and you're served a concoction you hardly recognize. Try to dissect the ingredients on your plate and make a mental estimate the calories – so you can compensate by eating less the next day. Of course, you don't have access to an accurate calorie chart, and even with one (without knowing the exact ingredients of the recipe) you would be lucky to come within 50 kcalories of the true total. In situations like this, don't waste your time trying to decide if that slice of bread you ate was 65 or 70 kcal, when your best guess for the main dish is 400 to 600 kcalories. What you should do is make a "ball-park" estimate.

To "ballpark," first you must know what elements are significant and then what approximate value you should assign to these elements. In other words, first you must know what foods or ingredients are significant, that you should even bother counting, and then you assign an approximate calorie value to these foods or ingredients using Table 32 – which is designed to help you make quick and reasonable estimates.

You Need Fiber

Fiber is an important part of a healthy diet. You need to consume fiber to assist your digestive system. According to the Harvard University School of Public Health, adequate fiber intake reduces the risk of developing various conditions, including heart disease, diabetes, diverticular disease, and constipation.

Three fibers that are eaten on a regular basis are cellulose, hemicellulose and pectin. Hemicellulose is found in the hulls of different grains like wheat; e.g., wheat bran is hemicellulose. Cellulose is the structural component of plants, and gives vegetables their familiar shape. Pectin is found most often in fruits, is soluble in water but non-digestible, and is usually referred to as "water-soluble fiber." The best fiber sources are:

- Whole-grain breads, whole-grain cereals, whole-wheat pasta and brown rice contain a great deal of hemicellulose fiber.

- Fruits are pectin rich (the water-soluble fiber). The skin on fruits are loaded with phytonutrients and fiber. So do not peal an apple. Eat it with the skin on and get a fiber and nutrient boost.

- Most berries (such as bilberries, raspberries) have even more fiber than a comparable weight of most other fruit selections.

- Vegetables have lots of cellulose fiber. Again the skin is particularly high in fiber. When you eat a baked potato, eat it skin and all – everything – everything that is except the butter or sour cream.

91

- Peas and beans are high fiber foods that are also a complete protein when eaten with a whole grain food, or nuts, or seeds.
- Nuts and seeds add fiber to your diet.

When you eat fiber, in any of its forms, it simply passes straight through, untouched by but aiding your digestive system. Zero calories absorbed!

Adults should get a least 20 to 35 grams of dietary fiber per day. How much fiber is in the foods you eat? An apple has about 3 grams of fiber, a orange has 2 grams, a tomato has 2 grams of fiber, broccoli holds 2 grams per 100 g, lima beans contain 4 grams of fiber per 100 g, oat meal has 10 grams per 100 g, whole-wheat cereal holds 10 grams per 100 g, and one slice of whole-wheat bread contains about 2 grams of fiber.

Water, Water Everywhere

The average adult female body is about 52 percent water, while the average adult male is approximately 63 percent water. If you are average, everyday you lose about 2500 mL of water when you breathe, perspire, and excrete waste. Because water is needed for almost every biochemical and physiologic process in your body, to maintain your body's water balance you must replace this lost water. (The water in your body is said to be balanced, when your water intake from all sources equals your loss of water.)

Typically, the food you eat every day contains about 750 mL of mostly concealed water. When you metabolize the food you eat, you create another 250 mL of water. That leaves about 1500 mL that must be replaced by the liquids you drink – more when you exercise. It appears, therefore, that the long-established wisdom advocating that you drink eight glasses of water per day (or any healthy beverage such as tea or fruit juice) is not far from the mark.

Use Salt Sparingly

Sodium and sodium chloride (salt) normally occur in small quantities in many natural foods. Salt and sodium-containing ingredients are also frequently found in high amounts in processed foods, such as canned soup and baked goods. People also add salt during food preparation and to the food they eat. Although sodium plays an important role in your body, many studies have demonstrated that high sodium intake is also associated with high blood pressure. In your body, sodium retains water expanding blood volume which in turn raises blood pressure. Moreover, although some questions remain, evidence suggests that many adults who are predisposed to high blood pressure (for example having a parent who has high blood pressure) can reduce their chances of developing high blood pressure by consuming less sodium.

Most Americans consume too much sodium. The U.S. Department of Health and Human Services and the Department of Agriculture Dietary Guidelines recommend that healthy adults **limit sodium intake to 2,400 mg per day.** (Note that one level teaspoon of salt contains about 2,300 mg of sodium.) Individuals who have high blood pressure and are also salt sensitive are frequently advised to limit their sodium intake even further.

Not Too Much Sugar

Sugars are carbohydrates that come in many forms. Sugar is found naturally in fruits, some vegetables, milk, breads, cereals and grains, and is often added to foods during processing, preparation and when eating. Added sugar and naturally occurring sugars are chemically identical and your body cannot distinguish between them. Cake, cookies, candy and many soft drinks contain large amounts of added sugar that supply a large number of "nutritionally-empty calories." Only very active people with high calorie needs can afford to consume any quantity of these sugar-laden foods. **Sugar should be used sparingly** by people with low calorie needs and in moderation by most other healthy adults. (Contrary to what many believe, the latest scientific evidence seems to indicate diets high in sugar do not cause diabetes. Rather, scientific evidence indicates that adult-onset diabetes occurs most often in those who are overweight.)

Common-Sense Nutrition

1) Know your daily caloric allowance whether you are trying to maintain your weight or are on a reducing diet.

2) Eat a variety of foods within your caloric allowance, and consult the Basic Food Groups to shape your eating patterns. Try to choose the proper quantity from each food group.

3) Try not to consume foods containing partially-hydrogenated vegetable oil because they are high in trans fats. This includes commercially prepared baked goods, snack foods, and processed foods, including most fast foods.

4) Limit your intake of saturated fats. Eat meat less often and fish and poultry more often, and use fat-free milk and milk products.

5) When possible, select fresh and natural foods and whole-grain products, and avoid chemical preservatives and additives, artificial and imitation foods, refined and processed foods, and foods that are mostly "nutritionally-empty calories."

6) **Eat nutritionally-dense foods** rather than calorie-dense foods.
7) **Take a daily multi-vitamin/mineral supplement.**
8) Before you buy, **read and understand the labels on food packages.**

Eat Slowly

One final important point, try to **eat slowly**. This is especially vital if you are on a diet, trying to lose weight. If you are someone who eats fast, who finishes before everyone else at the table, you are not giving yourself a chance to feel full. While everyone else is still eating, you either sit there and pick, or you have seconds, taking in extra calories you could avoid if you would just slow down. To slow down, try eating smaller mouthfuls, try chewing your food more thoroughly, and try talking more at the table.

Appendix B: EXERCISE

Many of us exist largely through mental efforts - by our wits and skill. All the advances of modern technology – from washing machines to automobiles to computers – have made life physically much less demanding. For most people, the common tasks of living and working no longer provide enough exercise to develop and maintain cardiovascular and respiratory fitness and good muscle tone. With any luck we can go for weeks without working up a good sweat or drawing a deep breath! Our bodies, however, are virtually identical to that of primitive humans who survived through physical efforts – by strength and stamina.

In fact, the bodies we inherited are just not built to be immobile and passive. The sad fact, however, is that after years of education and information programs by government agencies, medical associations and insurance companies, relatively few Americans engage in regular planned exercise – despite the reality that we need to be active to keep our systems working efficiently and rid ourselves of emotional tension. Moreover, exercise burns calories, speeds up your metabolism and is an invaluable part of any weight control program. There are two ways to become more physically active: First, increase the physical activity in your daily life; and second, start on a regular exercise program. Better still would be a combination of both.

Be More Active Every Day

Before we address exercise programs, here are some ways you can increase physical activity in your daily routine:

1) Change your attitude toward the occasional "bothersome" physical tasks that you encounter in daily living. Consider anytime you have to lift, bend, reach, walk as an opportunity to burn additional calories and as an extension of your formal workout.

2) Look for opportunities to walk, such as walking up stairs (two at a time if you can) rather than using an elevator, walking to a local store rather than driving, walking the course if you play golf, and mowing your lawn. At work stand up and stretch two or three times a day, read standing up, etcetera.

3) Engage in leisure activities such as dancing, bowling and gardening as often as you can. They can be enjoyable and provide added exercise.

Each of these daily activities taken alone may not seem like much, but done every day for many years they can add up to a substantial number of extra calories burned.

How Many Calories Do You Burn?

Table 33 on the next page shows the number of calories burned per hour for various activities. Although the data in the table are from reliable sources, you may find that some of the values are slightly different than those in other books. There are several reasons for this. First, the intensity of the activity being measured may actually vary (for instance handball can be played at many different levels – with a different number of calories burned at each level). Then the number of calories burned by same-weight individuals engaged in the same activity does vary somewhat; and finally measurement techniques and data collection accuracy vary slightly from laboratory to laboratory. The best one can do, therefore, is arrive at an average from the available data, which often requires judgment and compromise. More important, notice that the calories expended for a given activity depends on your weight. Good news: **For any activity, the more you weigh the more calories you burn!**

<u>Example:</u> Determine the number of kcalories burned by a 86 kg man (or woman) who walks 11 kilometers in two hours.

First calculate the person's walking speed = 11 km / 2 hours = 5.5 kph. Because 86 kg is not listed in Table 33, we use the neighboring value of 90 kg. Then from Table 33, we find walking at 5.5 kph, a 90 kg person burns 392 kcalories per hour. Thus, in two hours a 90-kg person would burn 2 x 392 = 784 kcal.

But from this we must subtract the number of kcalories a 90 kg person would have used anyway if, instead of walking, he or she just sat for the two hours. From Table 33 this amounts to 115 kcal per hour, or 230 kcalories in two hours. Then the net energy a 90 kg person would expend walking (over and above just sitting) totals 784 – 230 = 554 kcalories.

However, the individual in this example weighs 86 kg and would expend proportionately fewer calories than a 90 kg person: 554 x 86/90 = <u>529 kcal</u>

Types of Exercise

Simply stated there are **three basic types of exercise: aerobic, stretching, and strengthening**.

Aerobic exercises (also called "cardio") condition your cardiovascular system. Aerobic exercises, such as jogging, swimming, cycling, brisk walking, skipping rope, and many others, are typically deep breathing and continuous, with rhythmic and repetitive contractions of your large muscle groups. The trait most aerobic exercises have in common is that they make you work hard and require you to process a great deal of oxygen.

Activity	Weight (kg)								
	50	60	70	80	90	100	110	120	130
Aerobics (dance)	450	540	630	720	810	900	990	1080	1170
Basketball	350	420	490	560	630	700	770	840	910
Bicycling (20 kph)	400	479	559	639	719	799	879	959	1039
Cycling (stationary)	350	420	490	560	630	700	770	840	910
Calisthenics	313	375	438	500	563	625	688	750	813
Cricket	250	300	350	400	450	500	550	600	650
Dancing	229	275	321	366	412	458	504	550	595
Football	376	451	526	602	677	752	827	902	978
Golf (pulling cart)	248	297	347	396	446	495	545	594	644
Golf (riding cart)	174	209	244	278	313	348	383	418	452
Handball	335	402	469	536	603	670	737	804	871
Hiking	294	352	411	470	528	587	646	704	763
Hockey (ice/field)	394	473	552	630	709	788	867	946	1024
Horseback riding	197	236	276	315	355	394	433	473	512
Jogging (12 kph)	624	748	873	998	1122	1247	1372	1496	1621
Mowing lawn	275	329	384	439	494	549	604	659	714
Raking leaves	301	361	421	482	542	602	662	722	783
Rowing (moderate)	349	418	488	558	627	697	767	836	906
Sitting	64	77	90	102	115	128	141	154	166
Skating	349	418	488	558	627	697	767	836	906
Skiing (+country)	399	479	559	638	718	798	878	958	1037
Skiing (downhill)	303	363	424	484	545	605	666	726	787
Skipping rope	419	503	587	670	754	838	922	1006	1089
Squash	335	402	469	536	603	670	737	804	871
Swimming laps	404	484	565	646	726	807	888	968	1049
Tennis (singles)	294	352	411	470	528	587	646	704	763
Tennis (doubles)	223	267	312	356	401	445	490	534	579
Walking (4.8 kph)	178	214	249	285	320	356	392	427	463
Walking (5.5 kph)	218	262	305	349	392	436	480	523	567
Walking (6.5 kph)	277	332	388	443	499	554	609	665	720

Table 33: Calories Burned vs. Activity

In fact, aerobic is a word derived from the Greek, meaning "with oxygen." Aerobic activities use oxygen to produce energy. The main goal of an aerobic exercise program is to increase the rate which your body can process oxygen, i.e., increase VO_{2max}. A well-conditioned person with efficient lungs and a strong heart can pump large volumes of blood, can breathe large volumes of air, and via the blood circulatory system effectively transport the oxygen in the air they breathe to all parts of their body.

During aerobic exercise, the large muscles of the body continuously flood the heart with a great deal of blood; the heart beats faster; blood flow rate increases; and the lungs transport large quantities of oxygen to the blood. Regular exercise of this type "trains" the heart to pump more blood with less effort. Aerobic exercise improves the circulatory system by developing more elastic arteries and by creating peripheral or extra blood paths to the heart; and aerobic exercise strengthens the muscles of respiration increasing the volume of oxygen that can be processed within a given time. Done regularly, aerobic exercises improve stamina and endurance, and most importantly promote what should be your central exercise goal – cardiovascular fitness. For if your cardiovascular system is not in shape, you're not in shape – no matter how many push-ups or crunches you can do! In net, aerobic exercises develop a powerful heart, an effective circulatory system and efficient lungs.

Aerobic exercises can be further subdivided according to how strenuous they are and how well they condition the heart and lungs. (Note, there are exercises other than those shown that could be included in the groupings that follow.)

Group A: Bicycling, Cross-country skiing, Dancing (aerobic), Hiking in rugged terrain, Ice Hockey, Jogging, Jogging in place, Rowing, Skipping rope, Stair climbing, and Stationary cycling.

Group B: Basketball, Field Hockey, Calisthenics, Handball, Racquetball, Skiing (downhill), Soccer, Squash, Tennis (singles), Volleyball, and Walking (briskly).

Group C: Badminton, Baseball, Bowling, Croquet, Dancing, Gardening, Golf (carrying or pulling clubs), Horseback riding, Housework, Ping-pong, Shuffleboard, Softball, Tennis (doubles) and Walking (moderate to leisurely).

The vigorous exercises in Group A are intended for those already in good condition who want to further strengthen their heart and lungs and improve their aerobic capacity. The moderate exercises in Group B are not as demanding as those in Group A, but they are nevertheless good choices and can condition your heart and lungs. The exercises in Group C are actually not aerobic because they are either low intensity or not continuous, or both, but they still can be beneficial in that they improve muscle tone and coordination, relieve tension and burn some calories. (Note that some exercises in one group if done vigorously could easily be as demanding as those in the next higher grouping. For instance, a very intense game of squash could easily move it from the Group B to the Group A category.)

Stretching-type exercises such as yoga, tai chi, Pilates and to a lesser extent calisthenics can improve your flexibility – and some of the exercises can make you somewhat stronger.

As you age you inevitably start to loose flexibility. Your gait becomes stiffer; you can't stand quite as upright as you used to; it becomes tougher to bend over; and you have difficulty turning your neck. Regardless of your age, however, stretching can make you more flexible, less injury prone, and can reduce the pain and discomfort associated with tight muscles and shortened tendons. Realize, however, that stretching exercises do not condition your heart and lungs. Stretching exercises are fine as long as they are performed in addition to rather than in place of an aerobic exercise.

Most experts do recommend stretching before and after an aerobic or strength routine. However, never stretch cold muscles and always do some form of warm up prior to stretching. Stretch slowly and hold gently. You should stretch to the point of feeling a mild pull, but you should never feel pain. And **when you stretch – do not bounce**.

Muscle building and strengthening exercises, e.g., weight lifting, use of the machines found in fitness centers and isometrics.

Once more, as you age you loose muscle mass, your bone density decreases and you lose strength. Exercises like weight lifting strengthen your muscles, bones and joints. Strengthening exercises also reduce your risk of developing osteoporosis, a severe bone-loss disease, which can lead to easily fractured bones and all the complications that often follow. Strong muscles not only allow you to lift a sleepy four-year old out of a car without difficulty and lug groceries up to a second floor apartment, but as with increased flexibility, strong muscles also make you less injury prone.

Moreover, because muscle uses many more calories than fat, **when you replace fat with muscle, your metabolism actually speeds up**. In net, strengthening exercises are beneficial and should be a part of your fitness routine, but again they should be performed in addition to an aerobic exercise because alone they cannot condition your heart and lungs.

Select the Right Exercise

Selecting the right fitness exercise is the key to a successful conditioning program. You should try to pick an activity (or activities) you will enjoy. Factors to consider in choosing your activity
are: your medical condition, your age, your fitness level, your exercise goals, your daily and overall schedule, do you prefer to exercise outdoors or indoors, to exercise alone or with others, and how much money you are prepared to spend. You may decide to concentrate on one activity such as squash, or you may choose to walk briskly some days and lift weights on other days. Incidentally, three to five days of a vigorous aerobic exercise plus two days of either strength or flexibility exercises per week is a good combination. Whatever you settle on make sure it is an activity (or activities) that can be done regularly and that you enjoy.

Your Medical Condition: If you have a medical condition such as a heart problem, diabetes, osteoporosis, etcetera, or if you are a female who is pregnant or breast-feeding, you should proceed with caution, and be sure to talk to your doctor before you start any exercise activity.

Your Age: The age-dependent guidelines for how to proceed are as follows:

Ages 20-29: Assuming a clean bill of health from a medical exam, young men and women – unless badly overweight – can usually start an exercise program immediately.

Ages 30-39: The precautions here are the same as for the 20-29 year-old age group except that the medical checkup should also include a resting EKG.

Ages 40-59: Those in this age category should proceed with still more care by having an exercising or stress-type EKG as part of their medical exam.

Ages 60-up: The medical checkup is the same as for the 40-59 year old group. (Unless one has been physically active for a number of years, most physicians feel that at this age exercise should be limited to walking and moderate flexibility and/or strengthening exercises to improve muscle tone.)

Your Fitness Level: If you have been inactive for some time, rather than starting with one of the more strenuous exercises, **beginners of all ages should initially confine themselves to walking** until they can easily walk two miles at a brisk pace. When you reach this stage more strenuous exercises can be attempted if desired. Furthermore, some sports medicine physicians contend that **if you are badly overweight you should limit**

your exercise to walking at least until you have lost weight to the point where you are less than 25 percent overweight.

Your Exercise Goals: If you want to strengthen your heart and lungs, improve your aerobic capacity and burn a lot of calories select an aerobic activity from Group A or B. If you want to improve your flexibility select a stretching type exercise. And if you want to become physically stronger choose one of the strength-building exercises.

Your Schedule: Only you know what the demands are on your time from work, family and your social life. What is the best time of day for you? Which days of the week best fit your schedule? Of course, you must be open to rearranging your priorities to fit exercise into your daily life.

Outdoors or Indoors: f you decide to exercise outdoors you should also have an alternate indoor activity, an activity you can fall back on in bad weather. For instance, if you choose to jog outside early in the morning before work, you may want to purchase a treadmill for use at home on days when it is either too hot, too cold, or the weather is just bad.

Alone or with Others: On the plus side, an exercise partner can make exercise more enjoyable and can help you get going and keep going on days when you might otherwise quit. On the other hand, a partner probably means that you have the schedules of two busy people to contend with and plan around, which can at times actually hinder your workout.

How Much Are You Prepared to Spend: For many activities, you will need little or no special equipment. For instance, walking outside only requires comfortable shoes; whereas, joining and working out at a fitness center can be relatively expensive.

Aerobic Exercise: How Hard?

The central part of your exercise program should be an aerobic (or cardio) exercise done regularly. Additional stretching and strengthening exercises should be included as time allows – but never to the exclusion of the aerobic portion of your program.

An aerobic exercise program should be vigorous enough to condition your cardiovascular system but not so strenuous as to exceed safe limits. Some experts define safe as an exercise pace that is "comfortable." What they mean is that if, for instance, you are jogging or walking briskly you should be able to converse comfortably with a partner and that you should be breathing and feeling normally within ten minutes after you stop exercising. If not, you are exercising too vigorously. Other signs that you are pushing too hard include difficulty breathing, feeling faint, or feeling weak – during or after exercising. If you experience any of these symptoms, you are exercising too intensely and you should cut back.

Others prefer a more quantitative definition. They refer to the beneficial yet safe exercise region as the "Target-Training Zone," or TTZ, which is determined by monitoring your pulse. The idea is to raise your pulse through exercise to a specific range (the target-training zone) and hold it there for an extended period to obtain a cardiovascular benefit. On this concept rests the so-called heart-rated theory of exercise, which relies on heart rate (or pulse) to establish the proper exercise intensity.

Target-Training Zone

The **Target-Training Zone (TTZ) is a measure of aerobic exercise intensity**. Use the following to calculate your target-training zone:

1) Calculate your **Maximum heart rate** = 220 minus your Age. (Your maximum heart rate is the fastest your heart can beat, and you definitely must exercise well below this level.)

2) Compute your **Maximum heart rate reserve** = Maximum heart rate – Resting pulse.

3) Lastly, calculate your **TTZ** pulse = (Maximum heart rate reserve multiplied by Exercise Intensity level) + Resting pulse.

Walking Program

If your goal is to burn calories to control your weight and to improve your general health and fitness, walking is a wonderful exercise. Walking does have a downside. Because it is a relatively low-intensity exercise, to get a good workout you have to spend more time walking compared to many other high-intensity exercises.

If you are more than 50 years old, or have been sedentary for some time, it is best to start with a walking program that slowly but surely builds in intensity. If you walk hard enough, long enough and often enough, a walking workout can make you fit! A ten-week beginner's routine is shown in Table 34 on the following page.

The first session in week 1 starts cautiously with approximately three minutes of warm-up walking at a very easy pace of about 2.5 mph. Continue your warm up with two minutes of stretching. Then start walking more briskly, about 3.5 mph, but you should check your pulse and increase or decrease this to get your heart rate to a TTZ corresponding to about a 50 percent intensity level. After eight minutes of brisk walking, start your cool down by reducing your walking speed again to about 2.5 mph for three minutes. Conclude your session by doing about two minutes of stretching. The total workout time in the first week is 18 minutes per session. The only part that changes in succeeding weeks (2 through 10), is the brisk walking portion of the workout increases continually from 8 minutes in week 1 to 30 minutes in week 10.

Walk at least three days a week for ten weeks. If you find a week particularly tiring, backup to the previous week (or repeat the week) before continuing with the program. This is not a contest; you don't have to finish the program in ten weeks. Once you complete the ten-week program you can either stay with walking, or go to a more strenuous aerobic exercises.

If you decide to become a walker and want to improve, first go from walking three days a week to five days per week – at the same TTZ. To improve further, gradually increase your total workout time from 40 to 60 minutes. To improve even more, gradually increase your walking speed, and TTZ, so that your exercise intensity level approaches 60 percent. Another good way to increase the intensity of your walking workout is to include some hills in your route. Incidentally, as you would expect, walking over hilly terrain also burns more calories than walking on level ground. two of the days (nonconsecutive days) you don't walk, try to get in 20 minutes of strengthening exercises.

Because you will undoubtedly do most of your walking outside, you have to be aware of the weather forecast and have a backup plan for inclement weather. On bad-weather days, you could use an indoor walking site (like a mall, or an indoor track), walk on a treadmill, or do stretching or strength exercises instead of walking.

Week	Warm up (Minutes)		Brisk Walking (Minutes)	Cool down (Minutes)		Total Minutes per Session
	Walk	Stretch		Walk	Stretch	
1	3	2	8	3	2	18
2	3	2	10	3	2	20
3	3	2	12	3	2	22
4	3	2	14	3	2	24
5	3	2	16	3	2	26
6	3	2	18	3	2	28
7	3	2	20	3	2	30
8	3	2	23	3	2	33
9	3	2	26	3	2	36
10	3	2	30	3	2	40

Table 34: Walking Program for Beginners

Get a Pedometer and Step Out

Sedentary people only take about 2000 to 3000 steps a day. For the average person with a stride equal to about 2.5 feet (0.75 m), 2100 steps amounts to walking about one mile (1.6 km). A Harvard University study has shown that 6000 steps a day correlate with lower death rates in men, and that 8000 to 10000 step per day promote weight loss. And these health and weight management benefits don't oblige you to walk continuously until you accrue the required number of steps. Rather, all steps throughout the day to wherever and whenever count toward your daily total. (Some pedometers also show total "aerobic steps," correctly defined as those steps accumulated during at least 10 minutes of continuous walking at a rate of at least 60 steps per minute.) Because 10000 steps a day may not be achievable by some people, particularly by those who are elderly, sedentary, or who have chronic diseases, rather than insisting on a blanket 10000 steps per day, a stepping goal should be based on an individual's baseline steps plus an increment of additional steps. (Your baseline being the number of steps taken in an average day.)

A pedometer keeps track of your steps. And a study by the American College of Sports Medicine found that participants who used pedometers were motivated to add about 2000 steps to their daily routine. To start a stepping program, buy a pedometer. Wear the pedometer for a week and determine the number of steps you take on an average day. This is your baseline. Then add the equivalent of half an hour of walking to your day, or roughly 2500 extra steps per day. For example, consider a man who wears a pedometer and notes that on an average day he accumulates 3500 steps. His goal should be to add the equivalent of a half hour of walking to his day, or roughly 2500 more steps per day, for a daily total of 6000 steps.

There are many little ways to add steps to your day, such as taking stairs rather than an elevator, parking further from your destination, pacing as you talk on the telephone, marching-in-place for a minute once every hour – and of course taking short walks whenever you can. So buy a pedometer – get off the couch and step out for your health!

Jogging Program

If you are in reasonably good condition, have completed the "Walking Program for Beginners," or have been walking regularly, and have medical clearance, you can start a jogging program. Try to get your pulse into your TTZ but don't overdue it. Gradually, over time, increase both the intensity and distance of your jogging routine. However, if you don't have the physical makeup to do both, always choose endurance over intensity; i.e., choose distance rather than speed, choose to jog longer rather than faster.

The first session (in week 1) starts with approximately five minutes of warm-up walking at an easy pace of about 4 kph. Continue your warm up with two minutes of stretching. Then start walking more briskly, about 6 kph, but check your pulse and increase or decrease this to get your heart rate close to a TTZ that is roughly consistent with a 45 percent intensity level. After five minutes of brisk walking, jog for three minutes at a slightly higher heart rate, corresponding to about a 55 percent intensity level. Follow this with another five minutes of brisk walking and a three-minute jog. Cool down by walking again but now at an easy speed of about 4 kph for three minutes. Conclude your session by doing about two minutes of stretching. The total workout time in week 1 is 26 minutes per session. In weeks 2 through 13 (not covered in this eBook), the time allotted to brisk walking decreases as the jogging time gradually increases.

Jog at least three days a week for 13 weeks. Again, if you find a week particularly tiring, backup to the previous week (or repeat the week) before continuing with the program. Once you complete the program, if you want to improve, first go from jogging three days per week to five days per week – at the same TTZ. To improve further gradually increase your total workout time from 30 to 60 minutes. To improve even more, gradually increase your jogging speed, and TTZ, so that your exercise intensity level approaches 65 percent. Another good way to increase the intensity of your jogging workout is to try to include some hills in your workout. On the two days you don't walk, try to get in 20 minutes of strengthening exercises (see below).

Because you will undoubtedly do most of your jogging outside, again you have to be aware of your local weather forecast and have a contingency plan for inclement weather. On bad-weather days, you might use an indoor track, try an alternate exercise like jogging on a treadmill, or do stretching or strength exercises.

As always, stop exercising immediately if you experience tightness or pain in your chest, become lightheaded or dizzy, are severely breathless, lose muscle control or are nauseous. These are warning signs of over-exertion and you definitely should lower your exercise-intensity level. If you experience these symptoms, it's also a good idea to seek medical attention. Be aware that the pounding your body gets from jogging usually takes its toll over time. Many joggers have recurring, nagging injuries, particularly to their legs and feet. If you begin to suffer chronic injuries, remember there are other high-intensity aerobic exercises for which your body might be better suited. At that point, you might consider switching to cycling, a rowing machine, etcetera. Before abandoning jogging altogether, however, you might want to cut back, and only jog two days per week and try another high-intensity, non-impact exercise the other three days of the week. Variety will also make your workout more enjoyable.

Strength-Building Programs

As good as aerobic exercises are, they contribute little to building upper-body strength. If you are a beginner interested in strength training it's probably worthwhile to start by joining a health club, where you can get professional instruction on the proper use of exercise equipment, from dumbbells to rowing machines, and where you can compare different exercise routines. Another possibility is to hire a personal trainer for a couple of sessions to get you started on a program personalized to your fitness level and to teach you correct exercise techniques.

Of all the many strength-building options, I personally prefer free weights (actually dumbbells) because they can be used at home. Working out at home has some significant advantages. First, your workout takes less time because you don't have to drive back and forth to a health club; second, you have the flexibility of dividing your workout into small time segments to fit your day, whenever you have time, and of course working out at home is certainly less expensive.

You can workout in a bedroom, basement, garage, attic – anywhere you have extra space. A set of variable (adjustable) weight dumbbells and a small weight bench don't take up much room and are all you need for a home-based gym. (Bear in mind, **knowledge and the discipline to work out regularly are far more important than fancy equipment**.) Before investing in a set of weights and a bench, however, it may still be worthwhile to start by joining a health club. At a health club you can get expert instruction on the use of free weights. And you may find that you actually prefer to workout at a club. But if you do decide to opt for the convenience of a home-based gym, that would be the time to purchase a pair of variable-weight dumbbells and a strong weight bench (that will not tip over) for home use. Rather than an entire set of weights, initially purchase just enough dumbbell weight so that you can do a military press five times.

The seven dumbbell exercises that follow comprise a total-body workout, suitable for beginners, that involve all the major muscle groups. When done consecutively without stopping a series of exercises is called a circuit. To start, use the same dumbbell weight for all the exercises, a

106

weight that allows you to do 10 to 15 repetitions of the most difficult exercise in the circuit. For the first week do one circuit per training session. Your goal should be two circuits per session, which should take you about 20 minutes (with a two to three-minute rest between circuits). When you are comfortable at this level you are ready to increase the dumbbell weight – but by no more than roughly 10 percent (or one pound minimum). Again, perform 10 to 15 repetitions of each exercise.

a) Bench Press: With your head and back on the bench, hold a dumbbell in each hand to the side of your shoulders, palms facing each other. Slowly raise the dumbbells extending your arms above your shoulders. Pause, then lower the dumbbells down to the starting position. The bench press primarily works your pectorals, triceps and deltoids.

b) One–Arm Dumbbell Row: Hold a dumbbell in your right hand, palm facing toward your right thigh. Stand to the right of your weight bench and place your left knee on the bench. Support yourself by putting your left hand on the bench. (Flex your right knee slightly and lean forward so your back is almost parallel to the floor.) Slowly pull your right arm up until your upper arm is parallel to the floor. (Keep your right arm close to your torso.) Pause and lower your right arm to the starting position. After you complete a set, stand to the left of the bench and repeat the exercise with the dumbbell in your left hand. Rows mainly work your latissimus dorsi and rhomboid muscles in your back.

c) Seated Shoulder Press: From a seated position, hold a dumbbell in each hand to the side of your shoulders, palms facing forward. Slowly raise the weights over your head until your arms are straight. Pause, then lower the dumbbells to the starting position . The shoulder press mainly exercises your deltoids, trapezius, triceps, latissimus dorsi and rhomboid muscles.

d) Curls for Biceps: Stand with a dumbbell in each hand, your arms hanging loosely, with your palms to the side your thighs and facing straight ahead. Keep your elbows tucked into your side and slowly lift the dumbbells until they are approximately shoulder high. Pause and lower the dumbbells to the starting position. Curls chiefly work your biceps.

e) Tricep Extension (or Kickback): With a dumbbell in your right hand, assume the same initial position as in the one-arm dumbbell row. Slowly move your right arm rearward until it is nearly parallel to the floor. Pause and then return the dumbbell to the starting position without bending your arm. After completing a set, stand to the left of the bench and repeat the exercise with the dumbbell in your left hand. This exercise mainly works your triceps.

f) Front Squats: Stand with a dumbbell in each hand, to the side of your shoulders, palms facing each other (inward). Slowly bend your knees and lower your body until your thighs are almost parallel to the floor. Try to keep your heels on the floor. Pause and gradually raise your body by straightening your knees. Squats work your gluteus, quadriceps and hamstrings.

g) Curls for Abs: This is not a weight lifting exercise but is a useful part of any routine. Lie face up on a floor mat with your hands folded over your chest and your legs bent. Keeping your feet flat on the mat, slowly curl your torso up and toward your thighs until your shoulder blades are off the mat. Pause, then return to the starting position. This exercise works your rectus abdominis muscles – your abs.

Remember to do about five minutes of aerobic and stretching exercises before and after your strength exercises, and to workout two to three (non-consecutive) days per week. Why non-consecutive days? Because strengthening exercises work a muscle until it's fatigued, and a day off is needed for muscles to recover, repair and rebuild. And remember to listen to your body to determine your level of exertion. Don't over do it!

A final word about breathing properly: Never hold your breath during weight training. This can cause your blood pressure to get dangerously high. Rather, breathe naturally and try to exhale during a lift.

More Strengthening Exercises

As your conditioning improves, you may want a more challenging workout. This can be accomplished in a number of ways. One method is to use two pairs of variable weight dumbbells, with a different weight loaded on each set of dumbbells. Now, you can more closely equalize the difficulty of the different exercises by using the lighter pair for harder exercises and the heavier pair of dumbbells for easier exercises. Yet another way to make your workout more demanding is to add one or more of the following exercises to your routine:

h) Dumbbell Fly: With your head and back on the bench, hold a dumbbell in each hand and fully extend your arms upward with your palms facing each other. Keeping your arms fully extended, slowly lower the dumbbells sideways to chest level. Pause, then return the dumbbells to the starting position. The dumbbell fly primarily trains your pectorals, triceps and deltoids.

i) Dumbbell Pullover: With your head and back on the bench, hold a dumbbell in each hand and fully extend your arms upward with your palms facing each other. Allow your arms to bend as you lower the dumbbells behind your head. Pause, then return the dumbbells to the starting position. The dumbbell pullover primarily works your triceps and deltoids.

j) <u>Standing Back Press</u>: Stand with your feet about 12 inches apart. Hold a dumbbell in each hand at shoulder height and slightly behind your shoulders, with your palms facing forward. Slowly raise the weights over your head until your arms are straight. Pause, then lower the dumbbells to the starting position. The shoulder press mainly works your deltoids, trapezius, triceps, latissimus dorsi and rhomboid muscles.

k) <u>Knee-Bend Kicks</u>: Sit on the floor and lean back supporting some of your weight on your forearms. Raise both heals about three inches off the floor. Flex and lift your right leg. Return your right leg to its starting position. Then do the flex and lift with your left leg. Repeat as often as you can. This floor exercise works your abdominals.

Still More Exercises

There are literally hundreds of other aerobic, flexibility and strengthening exercises. Too many to review here, but many are definitely worth considering. For instance, swimming laps in a pool provides an excellent low-impact aerobic workout that also builds strength. Of course, the disadvantage is that you need to join a fitness facility that has a pool. Some trainers think a good rowing machine, such as the Concept II, provides a great total-body workout. Others feel a workout on a stairclimber is hard to beat. All have advantages and disadvantages.

In fact, most trainers recommend that you modify your routine every few months to add variety. Some advocate alternating exercises every other session. For instance, if you jog and lift weights on alternate days, you avoid repeating movements on consecutive days. As bonus, you will also likely avoid the injuries that are often associated with repetitive motion.

If You Miss a Workout

Inevitably, you will miss some workouts. It may be due to a heavy work schedule, a minor illness, or an injury. If you are injured or ill, wait for the injury to heal, or for when you feel like yourself before resuming your exercise routine.

If you only miss a day or two, you can undoubtedly just pick up where you left off as if nothing happened. If you miss a week or more, however, you will probably have lost some of your fitness gains and might have to resume at a somewhat lower exercising-intensity level. This means that when you come back after missing some aerobic sessions, you might have to exercise at a slightly lower TTZ, or shorten the duration of your workout. And when you return after missing some strengthening sessions, you might want to reduce the weight you are lifting or reduce the number of repetitions.

Incidentally, physical fitness can be maintained only by regular workouts. If your exercise frequency drops to one day a week, half your fitness gains will be lost in 10 weeks. If exercise is stopped completely, virtually all your accumulated fitness benefits will be lost in five weeks! Therefore, if you want to keep that state of well-being, feeling better, looking better, it's important to make regular aerobic exercise part of your lifestyle.

Risks and Possible Problems

Certain situations may occur that indicate you may be doing too much, exercising too hard. For example, regardless of your pulse rate you should never be left completely breathless by your aerobic exercise. A good rule to remember is: **You are exercising too hard if you cannot carry on a conversation while you are jogging, cycling, etcetera**. A feeling of having worked hard is fine, sweating is good, but not a feeling of undo fatigue.

Perhaps the most frequent problems faced by exercisers are injuries of the joints and muscles: sprains and strains, knee pain, elbow pain, back pain, neck pain, shin splints and stress fractures. Most happen when you exercise too hard.

Potentially serious problems are signaled if you experience any of the following symptoms during or after exercise. The symptoms include but are not limited to any abnormal heart action, such as an irregular heart rhythm, pain or pressure in the middle of your chest, pain in an arm or your neck, dizziness, fainting or lightheadedness, severe exhaustion, sudden loss of coordination, or confusion. If any of these symptoms are experienced, stop exercising immediately and get medical help.

Avoiding Injury

My good friend and workout buddy, A.C. Kanaar, M.D., specialized in rehabilitation medicine but he also preached what he called "preventive medicine," that is avoiding injury by practicing a common-sense approach to exercise:

1) Have a medical checkup and then set realistic fitness goals.
2) Build up your exercise intensity gradually over many weeks, months.
3) After you eat a meal, wait two hours before exercising.
4) Buy good equipment suitable for your exercise routine.

5) Use safety and protective equipment when appropriate, such as helmet when you bicycle, and goggles when you play handball, squash or racquetball.

6) Don't exercise outside on very hot day or very cold days.

7) If you insist on working out in very hot or cold weather, always let someone know when and where you will be exercising and when you are planning to return.

8) If you are new to a gym or health club, attend an orientation session before you use any unfamiliar exercise equipment. Otherwise, read the operating instructions carefully and ask someone qualified for help.

9) For aerobic activities, warm up slowly to reach your TTZ and cool down slowly after you exercise.

10) Do not increase the difficulty of any activity (e.g., your walking or jogging distance, the amount of weight you lift) by more than 10 percent per week.

11) Jog on softer surfaces such as a level grass field, a dirt path, or a running track.

12) After exercising wait 30 minutes before eating.

13) As a final point, if you experience some early warning pain stop exercising.

Keep an Exercise Log

Individuals who keep a record of their exercise generally exercise more often and have more success over the long term. How should you go about this? Keep an exercise log. A sample Daily Exercise Log is shown in Table 35 on page 112.

An Effective Low-Cost Exercise

Want an effective, low-cost exercise program? If your goal is to control your weight, improve your general health and fitness, try walking every day combined with two nonconsecutive days of strength training.

Walking is an exercise that you can do anywhere, that you can do outdoors or indoors, that requires no special equipment other than a good well-fitting pair of walking shoes, and an exercise that you can do well into your old age. Walking does have a downside. Because it is a relatively low-intensity exercise, to get a good workout you have to spend more time walking compared to most high-intensity exercises.

As good as walking is it does not build upper-body strength. Strengthening exercises, on the other hand, add lean body tissue, i.e., muscle, which increases your basal metabolic rate and helps in your battle to control your weight. For a good low cost strength-building option, try working out at home – with dumbbells. Your workout will take less time because you don't have to drive back and forth to a fitness facility and of course working out at home is definitely less expensive than joining a health club.

In short, a comprehensive walking program and working out at home with dumbbells can be the foundation of a total-body workout that can lead to a lifetime of fitness and good health.

Day	Walking Distance	Time	Heart Rate	Strength Exercise	Weight	Reps	Sets
Wed 08/11	2.7 miles	45 min	122	Bench Press	10 lbs	12	2
	5522 steps			Rows	5 lbs	12	2
				Tricep Ex	–	–	–
				Press	10 lbs	12	2
				Curls	10 lbs	12	2
				Squats	15 lbs	10	1
				Abs	N/A	25	2

Table 35: Sample Exercise Log

Workout: Lose Weight & Be Healthy

If your goal is a chiseled body with washboard abs and the endurance and strength of a triathlon athlete, you're reading the wrong book. Sure the aerobic and strength routines outlined here will help you get in shape, control your weight and get somewhat stronger – but your body is not going to be transformed into the physique of a world-class athlete.

This chapter is about how you should workout to control your weight, feel good and stay healthy. And you're not going to get fit just because you join a fancy health club with lots of high-tech equipment – if you only workout once or twice a week, every other week. Joining a health club is great – if you use it consistently.

The words that describe our kind of workout are consistent, determined, steady, persistent, dogged, unswerving, gritty, single-minded. Get the point? In our kind of workout, you decide that you will workout at least five days a week; that an aerobic exercise will form the core of your workout, and that you will incorporate some strengthening exercises two days a week

After that, it doesn't matter exactly what exercises you choose, what equipment you use, or what facility you use. These are secondary factors. What matters most is that you exercise consistently. **To improve muscle tone and overall fitness, feel good and stay healthy, you should exercise at least five days per week, day after day, week after week, year after year – for as long as you are physically able.** Remember the key words: consistent, determined, steady, persistent, dogged, unswerving, gritty, single-minded. Consistent!

NoPaperPress eBooks and Paperbacks

100-Day Super Diet-1200 Cal*
100-Day Super Diet-1500 Cal*
100-Day No-Cooking Diet-1200 Cal*
100-Day No-Cooking Diet-1500 Cal*
90-Day Smart Diet-1200 Cal*
90-Day Smart Diet-1500 Cal*
90-Day No-Cooking Diet - 1200 Cal*
90-Day No-Cooking Diet - 1500 Cal*
90-Day Perfect Diet - 1200 Cal*
90-Day Perfect Diet - 1500 Cal*
60-Day Perfect Diet-1200 Cal*
60-Day Perfect Diet-1500 Cal*
50-Day Flex Diet-1200 Cal*
50-Day Flex Diet-1500 Cal*
30-Day Quick Diet - Women*
30-Day Quick Diet for Men*
30-Day No-Cooking Diet*
30-Day Diet - Women - Metric*
30-Day Diet for Men - Metric*
25 Day Easy Diet-1200 Cal*
25 Day Easy Diet-1500 Cal*
25-Day No-Cooking Diet
10-Day Express Diet
10-Day No-Cooking Diet*
7-Day Diet for Women*
7-Day Diet for Men*
7-Day No-Cooking Diets*
90-Day Gluten-Free Diet-1200 Cal*
90-Day Gluten-Free Diet-1500 Cal*
30-Day Gluten-Free Quick Diet*
30-Day Gluten-Free No-Cooking Diet*
7-Day Diet for Women - Metric*
7-Day Diet for Men - Metric
7-Day Gluten-Free Express Diet*
7-Day Gluten-Free No-Cooking Diet*
90-Day Vegetarian Diet-1200 Cal*
90-Day Vegetarian Diet-1500 Cal*
30-Day Vegetarian Diet*
7-Day Vegetarian Diet*
Weight Loss for Women*
Weight Loss for Women - Metric
Weight Loss for Women - UK
Weight Loss for Men*
Maximum Weight Loss - 1200 Cal*
Maximum Weight Loss - 1500 Cal*

Weight Loss for Men - Metric*
Maximum Weight Loss- 1200 Cal*
Maximum Weight Loss- 1500 Cal*
Weight Control - U.S. Edition*
Weight Control - Metric. Edition
Prof Weight Control Women - U.S.
Prof Weight Control Women - Metric
Prof Weight Control Men - U.S.
Prof Weight Control Men - Metric
Weight Maintenance - U.S. Ed*
Weight Maintenance - Metric. Ed*
Weight Maintenance - UK Ed
Weight Loss for Senior Men*
Weight Loss for Senior Women*
Eat Smart - U.S. Edition*
Eat Smart - Metric Edition
30-Day Mediterranean Diet
Exercise Smart - U.S. Edition*
Exercise Smart - Metric Edition
Exercise Smart - UK Edition*
Total Fitness - U.S. Edition
Total Fitness - Metric Edition
Total Fitness - UK Edition
Total Fitness for Women-U.S. Ed*
Total Fitness for Women - Metric
Total Fitness for Women - UK Ed
Total Fitness for Men - U.S. Ed*
Total Fitness for Men- Metric Ed*
Total Fitness for Men - UK Ed
Senior Fitness - U.S. Edition*
Senior Fitness - Metric Edition*
Senior Fitness - UK Edition*
Computer Diet - U.S. Edition*
Computer Diet - Metric Ed*
Reliable Weight Loss - U.S. Ed
101 Weight Loss Tips*
101 Healthy Eating Tips*
101 Lifelong Fitness Tips*
101 Weight Maintenance Tips
101 Weight Loss Recipes
101 GF Weight Loss Recipes
101 Veggie Weight Loss Recipes*
30-Day Mediterranean Diet*
90-Day Mediterranean Diet - 1200 Cal*
90-Day Mediterranean Diet - 1500 Cal*

* These titles are available as both ebooks and paperbacks. Our ebooks are sold by Amazon, Apple, Google, Barnes & Noble and Kobo, but our paperbacks are only sold by Amazon.

Vincent W. Antonetti, Ph.D. is an emeritus professor at Manhattan College. He is a weight control and fitness expert who has lectured on

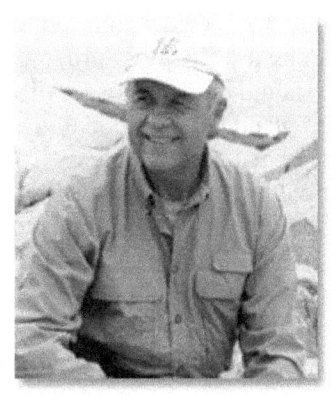

fitness at IBM Management and Professional Development classes and often speaks on fitness and weight control. Among his many publications is his highly regarded "The Equations Governing Weight Change in Human Beings," published in the prestigious *American Journal of Clinical Nutrition.* His paper was the first to develop an accurate equation to calculate weight loss. Dr. Antonetti's critically acclaimed book *The Computer Diet* was given Consumer Guide magazine's highest recommendation.

Recently, Dr. Antonetti coauthored "A Computational Tool to Simulate Energy Balance Components in Pharmacological Interventions," presented at Obesity Week 2016. He also co-authored (with Professor Diana Thomas) "Dynamic Modeling of Energy Expenditure to Estimate Dietary Energy Intake," Chapter 12 in Advances in the Assessment of Dietary Intake, published July 2017 by CRC Press. He is also the author or co-author of more than 100 eBooks and paperbacks. Many of Dr. Antonetti's books are listed at: www.nopaperpress.com.

Professor Antonetti is a life long exercise and nutrition enthusiast. Although a senior citizen he still maintains a vigorous physical fitness program - and has managed to maintain his weight to within 2 lbs (about one kg) of the 154 lbs (70 kg) it was when he graduated from college many years ago. He is now semi-retired and living in The Villages, Florida.

Disclaimer

This book offers general meal planning, nutrition and weight control information. It is not a medical manual and the author does not claim to be medically qualified. The material in this book is not intended to be a substitute for medical counseling. Everyone should have a medical checkup before beginning a weight loss program. Moreover, the physician conducting the medical exam should be made aware of and should approve the specific weight control program planned. Additionally, while the author and publisher have made every effort to ensure the accuracy of the information in this book, they make no representations or warranties regarding its accuracy or completeness. Further, neither the author nor publisher assume liability for any medical problems that might result from applying the methods in this book, or for any loss of profit, or any other commercial damages, including but not limited to special, incidental, consequential or other damages, and any such liability is hereby expressly disclaimed.